Movement IS Medicine
Volume III

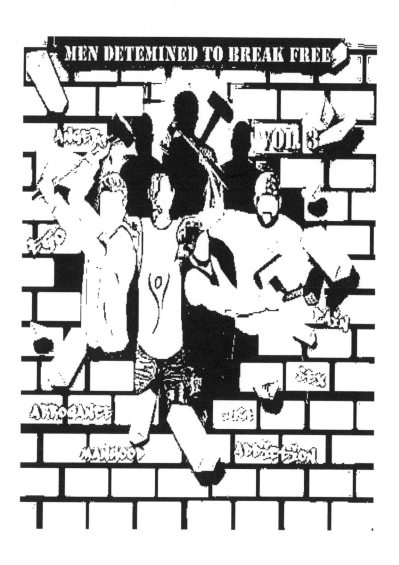

MEN DETEMINED TO BREAK FREE

VOL. 3

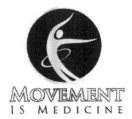

Movement IS Medicine Volume III Men Determined to Break Free

Copyright © 2016 by Movement IS Medicine

Creative Writing Editor Adia R. Edwards
Assistant Editor Adrienne Nolan-Owens
Cover Design Jean Bevins

Movement IS Medicine

Other books by Movement IS Medicine

Movement IS Medicine Anthology Volume I -
"Get Up and Move Something"

Movement IS Medicine Volume II -"Women Determined to Rise"

Movement IS Medicine Workbook and Journal

To my Little/Big brother Robert A. McKnight,
With love,

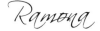

Movement IS Medicine

Table of Contents

~The Bridge~

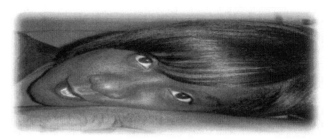

FOREWORD
Notes From Senior Editor

Adia Edwards

During the previous edition of the Movement is Medicine anthology series, I was a contributing writer and I remember feeling a mixture of anxiety, excitement and pride after I was given an amazing opportunity to share the most sacred and most vulnerable part of my self with the world—my personal story. I enthusiastically took pen to paper, fingers to keyboard and made a commitment to let down my guard, to be vulnerable and to write with sincerity and honesty in spite of how challenging that process was.

When Sister Ramona Gaines, a former student in one of my English classes, asked me to write about my struggles with adversity and my insurmountable determination as a child of two drug-addicted parents, I was immensely honored and instantly committed to the overall mission and the purpose behind Movement is Medicine. I was amazed at the trajectory and the scope of Pastor Ramona's vision. What started out as her courageously writing, blogging and sharing her personal weight loss journey with others via social media catapulted into a series of anthologies and other endeavors all committed to having individuals from all walks of life chronicle the demons, struggles, pitfalls, roadblocks and the detours which later manifested into accomplishments, achievements, successes, "aha moments" and ultimate personal victories.

Amazingly, a common thread that is visible throughout the different volumes and within each writer's story is the fact that each victory claimed resulted from our decisions to MOVE towards our God-given paths and sources of light rather than to wallow in self-destruction, misery, and self-sabotage and ultimate defeat. MOVEMENT is, in fact, the medicine, the secret "cure all" and the miraculous panacea- which each of us must take in order to walk into our destinies and to abandon the problems and issues which crippled us.

So, what can you expect from the men's edition of this inspirational anthology? Be ready to shed a tear, let out a chuckle, nod your head, let out sighs of relief and disbelief and to stop mid-reading, just to utter prayers of thanks, comfort and praise as each story serves as a reminder of God's grace and mercy.

We begin our collection with a tribute to an exemplary man of excellence, Mr. Kevin Lupton. Kevin Lupton passed away last March after battling cancer for 5 years. He served as an active and vital member and Deacon of Bright Side Baptist Church. In addition, he was a member of Kappa Alpha Psi Fraternity, a long-term dedicated employee of RR Donnelly and a loved, respected and admired member of the Lancaster Community. His tribute is a compilation of words from the hearts and minds of just a few of the many people with whom he had a direct and positive impact upon. These tributes from his closest family and friends, paint a portrait of a man who lived with honor, faith and commitment. Furthermore, his distinguished life and the impression that he made on this Earth exemplify a set of ideals which all of the male writers in this anthology have exhibited in one form or another. Specifically, by paying tribute to his life in the opening of this book, we also honor our Movement is Medicine writers' determination, conviction and the passion which has cemented their life purposes.

As an avid reader, creative writer and a person who seeks delight in connecting with individuals from all walks of life—I am amazed at the sheer diversity of thought, varied perspectives and unique experiences by the writers exhibits in this book. Conversely, they also share universal truths, mutual human emotions and similar struggles and challenges. You will also be shocked when you recognize the commonalities including insecurities, hurt, pain and vulnerabilities that the amazing men in our anthology share, as well. Too often we hold men up to unrealistic expectations and assume that they are invincible, unemotional and disconnected from their feelings. However, the stories told by the dynamic men in this collection reveal their emotions while shattering untrue myths of what it means to be a man in this complicated day and age.

I am thankful to each of the men in this anthology, our twelve disciples, for inviting us into their innermost sanctuaries- their personal lives. I am honored to be a part of this project and can't the wait for the day when I can gift my son (who is now 10-years-old) with his own copy of this life changing work of art. I am confident that he will learn valuable life lessons from this collection. Primarily, each of these stories speaks to the power of the human spirit to overcome adversity through faith, determination and the unwavering conviction to shout, "Mountains, move out of my way!"

Movement IS Medicine

Introduction: From the Desk of Founder and CEO

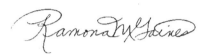 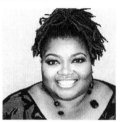

Anger, rage, sadness and hurt, those are all of the emotions that I felt all at one time on that day...

I must admit something from the onset of this writing, and that is this project was hard for me. Initially, when we announced in 2014 that we would be doing a men's book, my feelings were very different. I was excited and could not wait to step into the "Man Cave" and hear what was really on in the hearts and minds of men. We were going to hear their perspective and gain enlightenment and also understanding.

Many things happened to delay this project, and I am firm in my belief that we could not move forward until it was in Gods own timing.

Fast-forward to fall of 2015 and we began to kick the project around again and this time it kicked back and it began to come alive, it started to take shape and form. We were gaining momentum and I was bouncing off the walls with energy. But then that is when it happened, that voice on the inside of me said, "Are you going to help them after all that men have done to you?" I looked around to see where that voice was coming from because I didn't believe that it was coming from within me, but oh yes, it was and I had to sit with that. I began to question whether or not I had really ever gotten over all the things that had happened to me so many years ago? First off, my father was not an active part of my life, I was molested at four years old by a man, lost my mother to the man she married, was kidnapped and raped by a man, didn't have a relationship with my step-grandfather after my grandmother died, and I dealt with a number of failed romantic relationships that I expected to end with a marriage proposal. In so many areas of my life, I had experienced many heartbreaks and traumas at the hands of men. Some of them were by no choice of my own and others I went into with my eyes wide open.

So I asked God, "Are you really going to make me do this, do I really have to do this men's book?" God spoke back to me very clearly and told me that this project was not just about the men but it was about me as well. It was the tool He was using in this season for healing in my life, the lives' of the men telling their stories and all those who read it as well.

So once again I am back on the operating table with the Chief Surgeon cutting me open, taking out the parts of me that are hurting me. Bitter thoughts, broken dreams, rejection and so many other things that lurk in the crevasses and cavities of my mind. You know, the deep dark place that we don't want Him to touch? Yes, right there. That is where we are now. The good thing about that though is that God has the ability to cut and heal all at the same time when we give it to Him.

What I learned from the Men of Movement IS Medicine's Anthology has impacted my life greatly. I truly believed that it filled in the blanks in a lot of areas in my thinking about men in general. The lessons I took away included:

Lesson 1. Some men that were little boys sat in the window and waited for their fathers, as well. They created fantasies in their minds of when they would re-enter their lives and they often imagined what that reunion would be like. They fantasized about how happy they would be that their Dad/Father was present and when their fathers didn't show up, it hurt deeply. It hurt so much so that their emotions were packed tightly in a box with a "Do Not Enter" sign.

Lesson 2. Men hurt and act out in ways that we don't always understand. They also need to be loved, nurtured, and cared for in times of despair and trouble. Men aren't always strong and they don't always want to be. They need a safe place to cry and release to their hurts and to know that is okay to feel pain. They need to know they will not be seen as weak or lesser than a man in those moments.

Lesson 3. I'm smiling on the outside and hurting on the inside. Just as women need to be told that they are beautiful and loved, men need their egos stroked as well. Men should be told that they are handsome, needed and loved. For example when they get a nice haircut, make changes in their wardrobe or embark on a new venture. A compliment can go a long way for a man.

Lesson 4. The old hymn verse, we'll understand it better by and by," really does serve true. Some things we will just understand later on and we have to be okay with that.

Lesson 5. We must awaken the King in our men, our fathers, our brothers, sons, uncles and cousins as well as the men in our communities. They must be affirmed in their language just as we also affirm women and they must be consistently reminded that they too have greatness on the inside of them. We must consistently remind them that they have value and worth, what they bring to the table is important, it matters and it changes lives.

With all that being said, buckle up and enjoy the ride because the Men of Movement IS Medicine are Determined to BREAK FREE!

Tribute

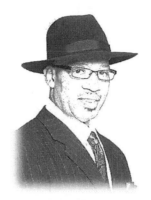

Kevin "Big Kev" Lupton

~A Man~

This tribute is dedicated to one of the first brothers that I met when I came to "the Ville." I've never met someone as equally massive, impressive, smart and grounded as Kevin Lupton affectionately known as "Big Kev." It is not that uncommon at this stage of my life to remember those who helped shape my college experience and my life, in general. "Big Kev," was one of those good brothers from Millersville University also known as, "the Ville," who did that. While we were originally brought together for academic purposes, I soon began to learn from his views, his perspectives and his wealth of knowledge. He also had a fun loving, contagious personality. I hope that everyone, when such people cross their paths, never take people like "Big Kev" for granted, but instead remember and embrace the moments and time spent together. I certainly never did, and never will.

"You carve your name on hearts, not tombstones. A legacy is etched into the minds of others and the stories they share with you."

Eric P. Jackson Millersville University Class of '83

~A Brother~

On a nice Spring Friday afternoon back in 1982, I visited a place that would change my life forever. I visited Millersville State University located outside of Lancaster, PA. This trip was set up for me to tour the university and also take an entrance exam. Millersville University's Head Basketball Coach Richard DeHart, who I had been speaking with for months, picked me up at the Lancaster Amtrak station and drove me out to campus. He asked Brian Wilson to be my host me for the weekend. Upon arriving on campus, we pulled up in front of the Student Memorial Center and I noticed a group of about 10-15 African American students (or should I say, I thought they were students) across the street sitting by the area near a building that I was informed housed the dining halls.

Coach DeHart got out of the car and immediately was greeted by the group. He introduced me as a prospective student for the upcoming Fall class. Many in the group were greeting me with chants of "Go somewhere else." Brian Wilson was in this group and immediately said that he was my host for the weekend. Also in the group was a Brother that was so big that he kind of like stuck out from the group. I noticed he did not say much but he did extend his hand to me and said in a deep base tone "You will enjoy Millersville should you decide to come, I am Kevin Lupton and I like it here." The big guy, the guy with the commanding speaking voice, the guy who introduced himself as Kevin Lupton from that day was always the same supportive person that I came to admire and respect in an enormous way. "Big Kev" as he was called was always a guy that you were excited to see.

"Big Kev's" proclivity for being a leader was not something that could be missed if you were in his company. Since our first meeting back on the nice Spring Day in 1982, I noticed that when Kevin spoke people listened. In a number of wonderful settings that I was able to enjoy Kevin would expound on many issues, which included the benefits of not eating white bread to the greatest fighters that came through North Philly to fight. He could hold court by just asking a question, and it would start some lively debates. By the way that group that I was welcomed by also include the likes of Joe Paige,

Steve Lewis, Harry Moody, Kevin Warner, aforementioned Brian Wilson, Mark Green, Andre Randall, Anthony "Deac" Walker, Fred Dukes and others, if my memory serves me right. Quite a group but Kevin Lupton stuck out. The guy that stuck out, the big guy with the massive Arms, the guy that looked like he was carrying suitcases under his Arms was actually one of the more compassionate guys that I have ever met. "Big Kev" always had time to talk with you about whatever ailed you.

Every year as Homecoming would arrive: the talk was always picking up "Big Kev," walking the yard with "Big Kev" and, having a place (hospitality suite) where we could "break bread" with "Big Kev." For years "Big Kev" and Sherry his wife entertained countless folks at their home when Millersville Alumni returned to the Lancaster area. There seemed to be endless projects that "Big Kev" was working on but, the thing was he would always listen to hear what you were doing. He would always ask about your family, wife, and kids but you were excited because he was listening. I remember the last Homecoming "Big Kev" attended and he was talking about some shirts that Calvin Johnson was hand painting to wear the next day. He talked about how Cal was going to get the shirts done and how he was always used to Cal's all night paint sessions when they were in school.

My life was changed definitely for the better by having a Fraternity Brother, friend, supportive African-American Male name Kevin Lupton in my Life.

During Kev's illness I visited him in the hospital, and it was very clear that he did not like being there. In "Big Kev" fashion he asked my wife Shanta and I if we indeed have driven from Maryland. When I said, "Yeah," he mentioned that he was happy to see us. Koy Stewart joined us; Kendall Banks and Deric Adger came also. Again and again I watched Big Kev greet people as he always has in my eyes, the way he greeted me way back on the Friday in Spring of '82. He was supportive. When we were there to support him he made sure that we knew that he cared.

When I think of "Big Kev," I am always reminded of the

Scripture that says, "For I consider that the sufferings of this present time are not worth comparing with the Glory that is to be revealed to us," (Romans 8:18 NIV)

Among men, the crowd of Fathers that we have become, Fraternity Brothers that have been entered into Bonds of lifelong friendship, Greeks, Nupes, Millersville Alumni, "Big Kev" stuck out.

Larry White Millersville University Class of '89

Kevin Lupton...during my early days and my pledge process that name rang out at the "Ville." My "Big Brothers" would say, "Oooo...you don't want big Kev to come," and when I saw him for the first time I understood why they said that. He was an imposing figure and someone who commanded any room he walked into. But truthfully, the "Big Kev" I met and got to know was the one who constantly had a smile on his face. He was the one who went out his way to encourage and help each brother out. He was the one who led the "Ville" Kappa's not just by his might but also with his warm personality, his kindness, and his genuine caring for his fellow man.

Derrick McCutchen Millersville University Class of '91

Movement IS Medicine

~A Father~

How do you quantify the true measure of a man? Well according to MLK's famous quote, "The ultimate measure of a man is not where he stands at times of challenge and convenience, but where he stands at times of challenge and controversy." According to author Michael Norton, "The true measure of a man is not what he dreams, but what he aspires to be, a dream is nothing without action." and to me, that is what my father was, a man of action.

I could go on for days about his, "Kevin Luptonisms," and famous one-liners, or how his presence commanded the room, even just by simply being present. My father was a lot of great things to a lot of great people, and to remember him they've used such adjectives as, hardworking, dedicated, loving, and God-fearing. Action is *MY* adjective. My Dad was a man of action, and it was his actions that built a legacy for his children to not only look up to, but also aspire for us to become.

It was my father's **ACTIONS** that allowed him to rise above the statistics of black males living in North Philadelphia. It was his **ACTIONS** that led him to seek higher education at Millersville University. It was his **ACTIONS** that provided his wife and children a stable home to be raised in, and from his **ACTIONS**, I have a blueprint for success, and an innate feeling of providing for my wife and children as well. My father was more to me than just "Dad." He was a living legend…a mythological being. And every day I was proud (and still am proud) to be his son. Death is never easy because it is permanent; however knowing that Kevin Lupton will forever live through our success as Lupton children, just makes reaching our goals and excelling that much sweeter. The true measure of a man is not what he dreams, but what he aspires to be…A dream is nothing without action." And that is what my father was, a man of action.

Marquise Lupton

What my Dad means to me...

My Dad and I had a very special relationship, and I think what made our relationship so unique was that we were so much alike. Being the only girl he always made me feel special. As a kid when he would come home from work I'd hide in the closet then jump out to hug him as he entered the house. We had countless "Daddy Daughter" days, we would sing oldies in the car together, and when he relaxed in his "Man Cave," I'd be close by in my toy room where he would occasionally peek in to see if I was all right. I remember everything my Dad and I did together from childhood to adulthood because we had the best times together. I was his "Piece Of."

My Dad was a hard worker and I always admired that, in fact I wanted to be just like him. I remember as a kid how he would leave for work in the early mornings then return before the sun went down. I remember how he would come home smelling like ink with a trunk full of groceries but still managed to cook a full course meal for us. My Dad provided for us and always let us knows the value of hard work. We weren't spoiled and we weren't rich but I remember always going on vacations during the summer and never being without. No matter how much my Dad worked he was always there for all of my dance recitals, school events, and sport events.

My Dad was in my opinion the perfect example of a man. He loved us and he loved my Mom. Although it wasn't always said it was always displayed because he did all he could for us.

Brittany Lupton

Battling with a terminal illness is something that words cannot describe and unless you have lived through it yourself, no one is in a position to make assumptions. When your doctor diagnoses you with a terminal illness and tells you your life expectancy based on the aggressiveness of the illness; that alone is enough to drive someone into a state of depression or just feel like giving up on life. I can truly say with pride *"NOT MY FATHER."* This man battled with stage four cancer for five years, and I can honestly say that I never heard him once complain or ask the Lord why did this have to be me. I have never witnessed such heart, courage, tenacity and a will to succeed from anyone other than my father. This is a man that loved his family so much and had such an unselfish heart that the doctors who were assigned to treat him were inspired as well as encouraged. My father had a never say die attitude and there was absolutely no quitting in this man. For me to express all of the love and admiration that I have for my father would take up more than half of the pages for the entire book. I am going to conclude by stating my father was a loving husband, father and a true inspiration to anyone that knew him or came in contact with him. He was a true man of God and will be greatly missed by hundreds of people.

Kevin Lupton Jr.

~A Husband~

Few events in life are as painful as the death of your spouse. You may be uncertain that you will survive this overwhelming loss. At times, you may be uncertain you even have the energy or desire to try to heal.

You are beginning a journey that is often frightening, overwhelming and sometimes lonely. My husband is everything to me and without him it's just not the same.

While words can never fully express how much someone means to us, language can still provide comfort, solace, hope and even inspiration following the death of a loved one. The way he treated me & the way I treated him, the way we took care of each other & our family, while he lived; that is so much more important than the idea that I will see him someday.

Lovingly Submitted,
Your wife Sherry Lupton

Movement IS Medicine

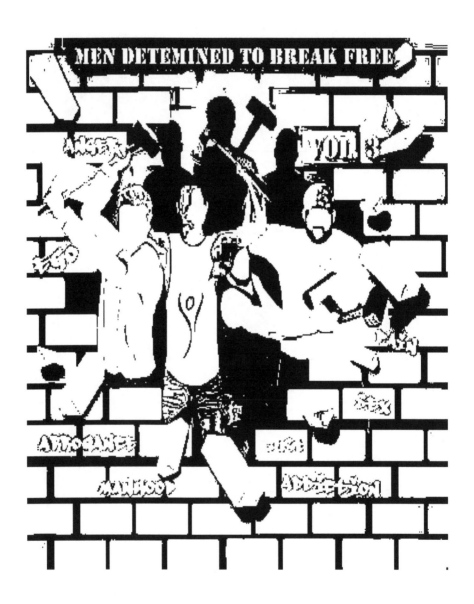

Chapter One

The Year I Became a Man!
By
David A. Rosario

YOU WILL NEVER GRADUATE FROM HERE!

These are the words that I will never forget as a young man. An insensitive lady, who was a nosy subordinate to the Vice Provost of the University, spoke these words to me. This was some time in the Spring of 1991. I was sitting awaiting my name to be called by the aforementioned Vice Provost. This meeting was for my University reinstatement. Previously, I had been instructed to send my application for reinstatement and supporting documentation to that office ahead of time. I clearly remember addressing my very personal package to the Vice Provost, but I guess this person decided to open it instead. So, here I am at the very young age of twenty-three, attempting my greatest comeback and being discouraged and dismissed by an enemy at the gate before I even had a chance to make a plea for my future.

The contents of my written package contained the detailed answer the question of 'How did I get here?' I felt totally disrespected knowing that a person to whom it was not intended, an inconsequential stranger, rudely violated the sensitive and personal recent history of my life! Additionally, this person didn't have the decency to keep it to herself. Even worse, she reduced my life into one sentence. The words, "You will never graduate from here", were now branded into my battle weary and impressionable mind. I was floored as if I was hit with a Muhammad Ali punch to the head. I knew that I had been wronged but I couldn't give this issue a priority status at this moment.

How did I get here?

This is a question that I had to seriously ponder during the nervous days leading up to my meeting in that office. I correctly concluded that this meeting would be the time for me to start getting honest with myself and the person that would be deciding my collegiate future. I was all out of excuses! My mind had all of the pieces to my 'honesty puzzle' whizzing about. It was difficult to gather my thoughts into tangible words. My embarrassing truths and my crazy sojourn were building up a wall of fear that was attacking my confessing tongue.

The battle in my mind was raging as my time was waning. It had been three and a half years since I had been enrolled in school and I had nothing to go back to at home. Those years gave me a glimpse of where my educationally stalled life was headed. And, as I waited, the unplanned daydream began. I started recalling and recounting in detail, how my college dropout life was born. Even though I had alluded to these events in my appeal package to return to school, the vivid memories kept opening up one after the other like an unhealed wound. My only piece of solace was that each time I recalled an event; it ended with going back to school as the only recourse for me.

The Descent!

The spiral started after a broken promise from a football coach at the university. I had not done what I was supposed to do academically in the Spring Semester. I had failed to achieve the required grade point average to move forward in school. The only option for me was summer sessions. I did not have the money so I went to the football offices and laid my petition before the coach that had recruited me. He told me to enroll in the courses that I needed and that the football team would pay for the classes to keep me eligible for the fall season. I was relieved and I did as I was instructed.

After two weeks of attending classes it was brought to my attention in a note handed to me by the disinterested professor, that payment had not been received and I must either make the payment or withdraw from the classes. When I brought this to the attention of the football coach, he told me that his promise to pay was no longer in the budget. That was all I heard from him. Everything else was blah, blah, blah. The tragic bottom line was that I was stuck. I walked away, angry, dejected and disillusioned. I didn't even bother to withdraw properly. That was a big mistake that would hurt me down the road.

I worked a couple of odd jobs in the university environment, intent on staying connected to school until I could figure out how to get back. This worked out well until the Spring of '89. During this time, I had a decent job and my own car complete with a monthly payment at the age of 20. I thought I had arrived! One day after work, I was on my way home when it happened. A car accident! I was hit by a teenaged driver and was hospitalized. My car was totaled and I needed a couple of months to heal. The college dream was over.

I had to move back home with my family and I was miserable. I wasn't in school, I wasn't working, I had no car, no money and I was immobile from the accident. My prospects were very low. My relationship with my girlfriend was hanging by a thread and I needed a lifeline because I was drowning.

Later that year, after litigation, I was awarded the princely sum of $4,000.00 as settlement for my life altering and disastrous car accident. I was 21 and the year was 1990. I was rich or so I thought. School was not on my radar, I needed to get out of my family home and get my own place, I needed a new job, I needed a new car, I needed to repair my relationship with my girlfriend. Little did I know that I needed way more than $4,000.00 to repair my broken physical life and there was no amount of money that could prepare me for the next leg of the journey that fate had in store for me.

The Fickle Finger of Fate!

By the Spring of 1990, my less than ideal decisions had taken shape. I was working 55 hours a week as an assistant manager at a Rent-A-Center. I was lifting refrigerators and delivering appliances to people that could barely afford the payments. Eventually I got hurt at this job by twisting my back during a delivery. Little did I know that this injury would be life's fickle finger of fate pointing in my direction. I reported this injury to the powers that be and they decided to deny my claim. This action on their part ignited my fury and my call to action. Little did I know that I would need all of my strength and desire because this was only the beginning of my journey back to school and I didn't even know it because I couldn't see it yet.

This injury kept me out of work for an extended period time and led to me seeking a lawyer to fight for a Workman's Compensation settlement. I never saw this part as a key in paying the back balance of my tuition that I owed to the University. But, that was not on my radar at that moment, I had to go through some more pain before that reality would come to pass.

At my second job, before my injury, I was a part time bouncer at a dirty little club patting down want to-be gangsters; looking for guns. There was already a formed a crew of bouncers employed at the club when I was hired. I never really connected to them because I could feel a vibe that I could not explain. It was obvious that they were a clique and were content on not having a new member, not that I wanted to be one anyway. One night, they approached me with an offer. These dudes were not only bouncers but also they were professional gigolos during the day and they thought that I would fit right in with their business model. I was flattered and all because I had always thought of myself as a handsome dude, but not to the level of a gigolo. Ha! These dudes were relentless in their recruitment of me. They had the game down to a science with the women that were soliciting for these types of services. The presentation and the money were very enticing but I turned them down and stayed content with risking my life for $100.00 per night. I quit that job within two weeks of the gigolo revelation. But the point of mentioning this part of my life is that it was relevant to my journey.

One night while at the club, the day before my injury at the first job, my apartment was burglarized. I came home to devastation and violation. Everything that I had earned and accumulated had been stolen. My black and brown leather jackets, my almost filled five-gallon water bottle/change jar, my prized stereo system and the punks even stole my cologne. I was beyond angry and emotional. It was 3 a.m. and I had worked both jobs so I had been gone for almost 20 hours; I did what anyone else would do, I called the police.

The two Caucasian male officers arrived at my home to survey and take a report. So, I thought! As I was attempting to get my mind right after working 20 straight hours, to tell these men behind the badge about my lost items, they seemed unconcerned about my loss. They began asking me questions about where is my mother, how am I able to afford this place, what do you do for a living, have you ever been arrested by police, do you do drugs, are you in a gang? I was furious. Of course, I didn't want to be arrested or killed in my burglarized home, so I kept my cool and refused to answer any questions beyond establishing that this is my residence. After I had done this, I politely asked the oath takers of service and protection to leave my home. The insult had indeed been added to the injury.

My girlfriend at the time was also my landlord's daughter. A couple of days later, after being injured at the first job, I called her dad out of courtesy to let him know what had happened and to see what could be done. Of course he told me that if I had Renter's Insurance then I could file a claim. I didn't have any, of course. Unbeknownst to him, his daughter and I were having our problems. She had graduated the year before from the same institution that we both went to and she was enjoying moderate success as a radio personality. I was no longer her educational, career-minded equal. I was now her long-hour working, two jobs having, no college degree, blue-collar grunt of a boyfriend at a time when she was on the radio flourishing in her career. I became a liability! The relationship failed soon after.

Now, after the injury, after the break up and after the break in, I was completely demoralized. I couldn't go to my old neighborhood because many of my old neighborhood friends were into things that would either get me into trouble with the law, shot or worse killed. I couldn't go to certain close family members because they had chosen substance abuse lifestyles that had rendered them null and void to the everyday world. I don't want gloss over this lightly. This was my big secret and my biggest embarrassment at this time in my life. Every key adult member of my immediate family at this time, except for my Grandmother, was a substance abuser. I was alone and dare I say-afraid.

The cherry on top of my disenfranchisement was that there was a rumor going around about the break-in at my apartment. The hurtful belief was that it was a close family member that robbed my home and stole my belongings. I tried with all my heart not to feed into this but it was hard not to. A few of the things that were stolen from me were not in plain sight and were only seen by a few folks that had visited me over the last year. This was a tough pill to swallow, but I prayed and let the Universe, Karma and Jesus deal with the matter. I had no more room on my plate to dig into this bitter meal.

I had quit one job, I was locked in litigation with another, I decided against enlisting in the Armed Forces and my money was very low. I was a mess. All I could do was muster some mental energy to make a desperate phone call to a trusted friend. When he answered the phone, I could only get a few words out of my mouth before, the mighty man that I thought I was burst into pitiful tears. After I gathered myself and explained my horrific journey, my friend on the other end only uttered a few lifesaving words to me, "What time will you get here!"

I sacrificed much of my material belongings and I headed up to West Chester, PA where my friend and fraternity brother resided and where I was disconnected from my college hopes. He had prepared a place for me in his humble apartment. It was here that I felt peace and healing. It was here that I was able to assess and pick up the pieces to my well-worn 21-year-old life.

Coincidentally, this was also the office location of my attorney that was assisting me with my workmen's compensation hearing. I mention him because it was this man that believed in me and structured a plan that would get me in position to realize a return to college. He urged me to sign over my settlement to him and he would help me. This was a huge act of faith on my part but I had one last strand of faith left and I gave it to him. Besides, I knew the poor decisions I had made with my earlier settlement from the car accident.

This wonderful man was Godsend. He called a client that had student rooms for rent and urged him to rent me a room to me with the understanding that he would not get paid until my case settled. By the way, there was no guarantee that I would win. The man still rented me a room. He called the University on my behalf, he sent them a letter of protection stating, that he would remit all outstanding fees owed when my case settled if they would consider my petition for reinstatement and allow me to register for Summer classes as well, if reinstated. He assisted me with an allowance each week and when my case eventually settled, he held true to his word, he paid all parties, he gave me a check for what was left and it was only later that I realized that he took no fee for his services. Mr. Goldman, wherever you are, I thank you from the bottom of my heart!

Onward.

The Day of Reckoning was now here. I had no more time to waste. It was my time to answer and atone. But my nerves were affecting me, I was afraid to have my truth to exposed to a stranger armed with a pen, pad and a ticket to my future. It was time to be a MAN!

As my name was called, I felt like a dead man walking the green mile toward my execution, instead of a remorseful and rehabilitated young man ready for his future. The reason I felt this way was because my honest answers, my truths, were poor decisions that reflected my immature character development at that time in my life. My sad reality at its foundation was this:

I was not in school partly because I was having too much fun,
I was not in school partly because I didn't do my part in the classroom.
I was not in school partly because a trusted athletic coach had lied me to.
I was not in school because I pledged a fraternity and decided that road trips, parties and visiting pledges at other schools were my top priority.
I was not in school because spending time chasing girls and one girl in particular was more important than my education.
I was not in school because of my poor choices and my lack of discipline.

At that moment, I knew that it was more important for me to recognize this and tell it to this decision maker before she told it to me. This was going to be the only way I would make it back to school for my second chance at success.

The Hits Keep Coming!

After successfully navigating the reinstatement process, I was granted a provisional admission status for Summer 1991. This determination contained the promise of full time admission in the Fall, if I successfully completed the 3 summer classes. I accepted that challenge and went full steam ahead! But, I had to address those three Summer classes that I did not withdraw from back in '88. My transcript was looking real shabby. I had 7; count them SEVEN F's on my transcript and a 1.4 GPA. That emotional decision that I made had cost me dearly. It took some serious research and committed communications to get in touch with those professors to confirm that I had not tested in their class and my attendance was only the first two weeks. Ultimately, I was able to get those three F's administratively withdrawn. And I had to repeat the other 4 classes to get those F's combined into one grade.

During the fall semester, I was beyond happy to be back in school on a full time basis in the nurturing environment of College. Although I was a 23 year- old sophomore, I felt like an 18-year-old freshman with a second chance. Everything was smooth; I was thoroughly immersed in my studies and believed I was on my way. Then the phone rang! A representative of Student Affairs that wanted to meet with me about my reinstatement application called me. I scheduled a time to attend. All I could think at this moment was, "what in the world is going on now?"

I nervously attended this meeting without a clue as to why I was being summoned. All of my affairs were in order and I was in a good headspace. And I had no clue as to why anyone in this office wanted to meet with me. Well, at this meeting I was informed that I answered a question on my application untruthfully and a Student Judiciary Session was required to address this matter. Furthermore, if the accusation were to be upheld, I could be faced with expulsion. I was floored. I was mad. I was indignant because I had been nothing but truthful and integrity filled at every step of the way.

I reviewed the item on the application that was in question, and it was some bull. The question was very ambiguous; it was constructed to be misleading. I don't remember the exact wording now, but it was something to the effect of have you ever or were you cited for... I answered NO on the application because I had never had any interaction with Student Affairs as it pertained to being disciplined. They maintained that back in 1986, when I was a freshman I was written up in the dorm for beer in my room. This was true but I never signed anything or had to attend any meeting. The Resident Assistant told me that it was no big deal and I treated as such and never thought twice about it. Honestly, I forgot all about it, it was 1986; 5 years ago, a whole lifetime ago and I didn't even drink! It was my roommate's stuff.

Now, after all of the changes that I had gone through to go back to school, here I was being faced with more adversity; a challenge to my integrity, another enemy at the gate, another obstacle in the way of my educational goals. Whew! I was given a date and time to appear. I was told to gather my supporting materials and then the matter would be addressed. This was September 1991, the second week back in school.

I needed to talk to the only person that would ease my spirit and give me wisdom to traverse this issue, my grandmother Marian. I went home that weekend to seek her out. When I arrived home, no one was around. Not my grandfather, my two uncles that lived there and not even my mother who frequented her childhood home as well. My grandmother was alone in her bedroom, writhing in pain. I tended to her needs as best I could, to comfort her. She was adamant about not wanting to go the hospital. I have always respected her to the utmost but this was a command that I found fault with. I pleaded with her to relent and allow me to call an ambulance. She was insistent on not going. I was stuck and no one was at home to assist me. So, I was also pissed that my elderly grandmother had not been afforded care from family. I prayed for guidance.

I made the most difficult phone call of my life. I called for an ambulance against the wishes of the woman that I loved as much as anyone else in the whole world. I was devastated to defy her but I knew in my heart that I was doing the right thing. As it turned out, it was the right thing to do and she was rushed into the first of two major surgeries. The second surgery that took place on October 12, 1991 turned out to be too much for her frail body and dire condition to handle. She was gone! The love of my life, my heart and soul gone from this Earthly plane at a time when I believed I needed her most.
I was devastated. I was rocked to my very core and I was filled with rage, depression and sadness all wrapped into one. To this day, I miss her.

How bad do you want it?
After laying my beloved grandmother to rest, after consoling my mother and being strong for my family, I went back to college to face another challenge, and that potentially contained more devastation. I was a zombie; I had no fight left in me. The university did not

35

grant me any more time to gather myself. They wanted their pound of flesh and they wanted it immediately, without an ounce of sensitivity attached to it. I met with a University Psychologist who happened to be a Fraternity Brother of mine. I trusted him and I laid my heart and situation out on the table for him to view in its rawest form. I had nothing left to give to anyone or anything else. I didn't care anymore.

Dr. Saddler was sent by God to be my angel in a time of great need. He asked me multiple questions and dialogued with me for hours. The main things I remembered from him were the pearls of wisdom that he imparted to me. He asked me, "How bad do you want it"? He told me, "The tassel is worth the hassle." And he told me that my grandmother would not have left me without knowing that I had everything I needed to get the job done. It was these words during our sessions that pulled me through emotionally. It was these sessions that kept me moving and improving. It was these sessions that gave me the strength to go forward with my fight with the University, to win my appeal, to take 96 credits in 2 1/2 years. I attended Fall, Spring and Summer classes nonstop until I graduated in the Fall of 1993. I even found time to play my beloved football again for the University in 1992 and 1993. I will always remember 1991 as the year I became a man!

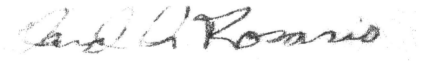

Movement IS Medicine

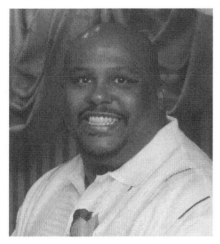

David A. Rosario was born and raised in Philadelphia, PA, to an African American Mother and Puerto Rican Father. This union allowed David to have a unique upbringing by having two very different families, experiencing two vibrant cultures and speaking English and Spanish.

After graduating from the renowned Central High School in Philadelphia, David attended West Chester University on scholarship for Football and Basketball. He graduated with a Bachelor of Arts in Communications and continuously pursues lifelong learning about Ancient African History. David is also an Entrepreneur, having started several successful businesses in Real Estate and Order Fulfillment.

David has spent parts of the last 20 years working in and around Philadelphia as an advocate for youths and families. He has worked in the School District of Philadelphia and the Mental Health Community over the years. He currently works with elementary school children that suffer with diagnosed behavioral challenges.

David is a champion of children and families in needy communities. He has been a volunteer football coach for the School District of Philadelphia. David has also volunteered with the Salvation Army and various community centers and churches. He is a proud member of Omega Psi Phi Fraternity and has served as President of His Graduate Chapter, Omega Xi.

David is married to a loving wife, Zara and has four beautiful children. Education and the pursuit of dreams are emphasized in the Rosario household.

David is a modern day "Renaissance Man" and spends his spare time writing songs, poetry and short stories as a hobby. This is the first time his work has been published.

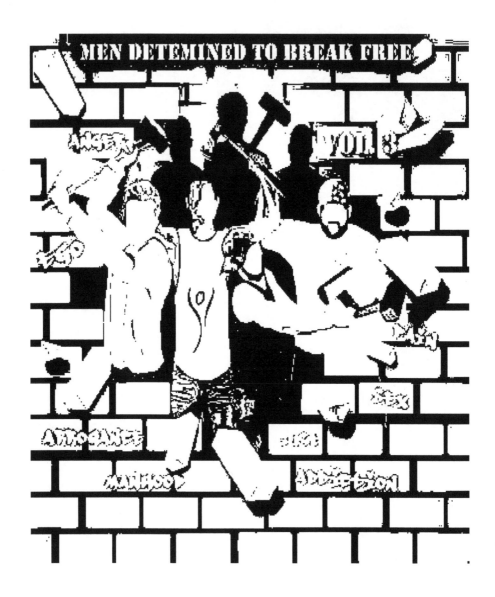

Chapter Two

To Dad

By

Weston C. Strader II

W Strader
God Bless!!
Matthew 7:14

Dear Dad,

Well here we are 22 years after your death. At the ripe age of 25 and about to graduate from college I had no idea of how and/or if your passing would impact my life. The reality is that you walked out the door of our apartment when I was 11 years old but had checked out on my sisters, your wife, and me many years prior. The later departure was driven by your one true love or the comfort only alcohol could provide you and it is for that reason I wonder if you were ever really there for me.

You are probably asking why I am writing and addressing your absence now? Where is this coming from? Well, I was approached to be involved in an incredible writing project that will ultimately attempt to provide spiritual motivation and inspiration to others. My first thought was to write a love letter to my children about the impacts of being raised fatherless and how I overcame those struggles. That would have been the easy route because I would not have had to deal with a bunch of emotions that I have not dealt with in a while. I am choosing a different route. If this is going to be inspirational, I need to share the depth of my disappointment and ultimately how and who were responsible for bringing me through it.

I want to first say I understand not all relationships work out and that you and mom were obviously better for divorcing. It should be noted, it's taken me a marriage, kids, and lots of maturing to have this outlook. As a child and even sometimes as a young adult, I can remember wishing you guys would have "toughed" it out and just "made it work" for us kids. But Dad, checking out totally on every emotional, financial, and spiritual level was totally irresponsible. For the life of me, I cannot understand how you could do that to your kids and a woman you shared three kids with.

You left us in a poor, economically depressed, suburb of Allentown, PA. And while Catasauqua may not have seemed like a bad area to most, we were one of a few black families in that entire northeast Pennsylvania community and racism, hate, and all that goes along with the two were dealt with on a regular basis. I remember fighting Jeff White on Easter Sunday because he had called my sisters "niggers". Yep, on the same day we were celebrating the most selfless and loving act of God, I was defending my sisters honor from the use of one of the most vile and nastiest words known to man. The neighborhood was laced with drugs as well. One of my best friends ended up with a serious drug problem and in rehab at a very young age. The guys used to smoke "pot" and make fun of me because I had no clue as to what that meant. What were you thinking? How could you leave three young kids and a wife in that environment?

Even if the environment had been better, I think about our material needs and how we did not grow up with much. I remember my mother having to always plead with you to pay child support – also known as the government's definition of the bare minimum for providing for your kids based on your salary; and you could not even do that consistently. Our need to eat and be clothed was very consistent. As a result of your failure in this department, my mother took filling this void seriously for her children's welfare was at stake. She worked hard, became a young executive at Xerox, and was able to provide most of our material needs on her own. I recall your inability to pay support getting so serious the authorities were going to lock you up, but my mother did not want to see the father of her children imprisoned and would not agree to move forward with the procedure for them to do so. Inconsistent is the best word to describe your ability to provide for us. I can recall birthdays and

Christmases without so much as a card. I know this had to be incredibly stressful for her. Aside from the day-to-day care she provided, she had little to no support from you and all I can do is shake my head. I look at my kids today and say if God forbid something ever happened between their mother and I, material needs are the last thing they would be thinking about. Those needs would categorically be met and I would also be doing everything in my power to fill their intangible needs.

Aside from the lack of material support, there was more pain and hurt that came from just a lack of your presence. For example, the fact that you were not present for one single swim meet, I remember swimming and having a spot picked out in the stands where I pictured you cheering for me as I swam. It never happened. Swimming is both a team and an individual sport. While at practice, you have a lot of time by yourself to think. I can remember countless hours practicing and thinking about our relationship or the lack there of. I truly think it was therapeutic as it allowed me a safe place to think and deal with the emotions and feelings of not having a relationship with you. While I did not realize it then, I was grieving your loss and preparing myself to move on without you.

I remember your sisters, Aunt Trish and Aunt Cathy, calling us and letting us know you were not doing well and that we should probably come see you as your days were clearly numbered. By this time in my life (1993), I had already dealt with losing you. To me, this was just the official closing of a chapter that had already been written. Aunt Trish and Aunt Cathy insisted that my sisters and I come to see you. I pushed back and said that I had already dealt with your loss and that I wanted my last memories of your physical manifestation to be one of you in good health. However I eventually gave into their requests to come see you. I never remember hearing you say you loved my sisters or me and figured this would provide you with that moment. If there was ever a time I would hear it, this was going to be the time. Heck, I was thinking maybe, just maybe, I could also get an apology for you not being there for us as kids.

Once again, this was wishful thinking. The same type of wishful thinking that I had as a kid when it was your turn to take us for the weekend and you would not show up. It was also the same type of wishful thinking I would have doing flip turns during some of my biggest swim meets thinking you would magically appear in the stands to cheer for me. Again, the same type of wishful thinking I had while driving home from high school graduation thinking you missed the ceremony because you got lost, only to arrive at the house and not see you there. You were in an alcoholic coma and barely coherent. None of what I hoped for transpired and my last and final memory will be of you hooked up to all those tubes, once again unable to deliver anything I needed. I obliged the family's wishes and cares for your sake and came to the hospital, not sure I would have made the same choice today.

Living in a heavily populated military area, I often hear military parents who lose children to combat say they find a certain degree of solace and comfort in knowing their children lost their lives "doing what they loved" and defending their country. I guess I can take a certain bit of this comfort knowing you lost your life wrapped in the arms of your one true love – alcohol.

I am 47 years old, live in Smithfield, Virginia, have two lovely children (Ethan and Evynne), am happily married to my soul mate (Billie) for almost 16 years and have been gainfully employed as a Senior Vice President with a reputable financial institution for the past 13 years. I am living a life better than I would have ever dreamed when I was a child. How did all this happen? The narrative of most kids in this situation typically includes a spiral out of control, possible drug use, and an almost certain life- long connection with the criminal justice system. None of which I have had to endure. Aside from an incredible mother who worked like heck to provide for us and keep my sisters on the straight and narrow, I was blessed to have a loving and generous family who stepped in and tried to fill the void left by your departure.

Uncle Skip, one of mom's older cousins, played a major part in teaching me to be a man. He loved the racetrack and a stray skirt sometimes distracted his eyes, but these imperfections did not consume him. He taught me through his actions and not merely his words. While there was an occasional lecture, he lived his life through actions rather than a bunch of meaningless words. While living with him and the Taylor clan, I learned the value of getting up and going to work every day. I saw first-hand how a man and woman in a loving relationship interacted. I saw how a man treated his queen, the woman he openly professed to love. I saw how he treated and loved his kids; how he took care of them materially and how he supported them spiritually and emotionally through his words and actions towards them.

While I only lived with him and Aunt Doris for two summers, they were two of the most profound for me as they played a significant part in shaping me into the man I am today. Uncle Skip exposed me to faith and not just any faith but a faith rooted deeply in the blood of the Lamb. His was a faith rooted deeply in the love and adoration for Jesus Christ. Again, he did the majority of this through his actions, but I can remember one brief lecture he gave me upon arriving to his house the first summer. He sat me down and explained the rules and expectations of living in his home. There was the normal stuff like cleaning up after myself and a small list of chores, but rule number one was attending church on Sunday morning. He said no matter how late I was up on Saturday night or what I thought was important on Sunday morning, I was to be in church. He also let me know that as a deacon, he sat in the pulpit and that he would know if and when I arrived. This rule was clear, firmly understood, and not something he would ever have to say twice. Little did I know the lesson I would learn from this rule. It taught me what it meant to be consistent and dedicated to something – no matter what. Over the two summers, I ultimately grew to understand that there was joy, peace, and comfort in a relationship with Jesus Christ.

The other thing I remember is hearing him sing while we were working. He was no Luther Vandross, but his singing ministered to me. His favorite hymn was Blessed Assurance. I could see a perfect peace come over him when he sang the chorus, "this is my story, this is my song, praising my savior all the day long". I could hear humility in his voice when he sang, "heir of salvation, purchase of God, born of His Spirit, washed in His blood." But most of all I could hear clarity, conviction, and comfort when I would hear him sing, "Perfect submission, all is at rest, I in my savior am happy and blest, Watching and waiting, looking above, filled with His goodness, lost in His love."

Dad, I learned that while a relationship with you is something I yearned for, a relationship with Christ is what I needed as He would provide me with Grace, Mercy, Peace and Comfort far beyond any of the things you could.

I think about the relationship I had with your mother and wonder how you could be so different from her. While she could not teach me anything about manhood, she was another tremendous influence on my life. This wonderful white woman showed me love, provided me with valuable life skills, and taught me invaluable lessons about the importance of family. She also taught me lessons about money. Not necessarily about investing but about saving and the importance of doing so to cover yourself in the event of a rainy day. She would always tell me to not let the money, "Burn a hole in my pocket." I can hear her saying it to me every time I tell my children the same.

She was an incredible cook and taught me how to do so. She did not see cooking as a chore but more of an act of love. She poured tender loving care into every meal she prepared. Good food was something people just came to expect from Grandma and it was because she cared so much about each and every meal she prepared. I carry that same mentality into the kitchen for every meal I prepare as well.

She also taught me about the importance of family. She was at every family event, never missed a birthday, Christmas, or Easter with a card, and always had time for a conversation or encouraging word through either a letter or a phone call. As an adult I grew to appreciate this and carry it with me today. It's so important to support those whom you love through thoughts, words, and deeds.

Like Uncle Skip, she too had an impact on my faith/spiritual development. After Grandpa Strader died in 1968, it probably would have been very easy for her to leave Bethel AME church for one that looked more like her, but she remained there. As a teenager attending that church with her, I could see she considered them her church family, she loved them, and they loved her back. I remember sitting next to her during service and hearing her sing. She had two favorite songs/hymns. The first is "His Eyes are on the Sparrow". There were three parts of this song that really stuck out to me; "why should I feel discouraged", "When Jesus is my portion", and "His eye is on the sparrow, and I know he watches me." These words coupled with the conviction she sang taught and confirmed a lesson I have carried with me through life. With Jesus as my portion, as my friend, it really doesn't matter how bad things look around me because he is a constant in my life and if He supplies all that the sparrow needs, surely He will do that for me.

Dad while this letter has expressed some heartfelt emotions and some disappointment that we have never really discussed there are a few key messages I need you to walk away with. Not having a relationship with you is one of the, if not the, biggest disappointment of my life. It denied me a true example with all its ups and down, perfections and imperfections of the wisdom and love an earthly father shows his children. That is something ONLY YOU could have taught me. And while I was surrounded by great family members, some mentioned and many not mentioned, that provided me with a lot of guidance on life, that is something that could never replace the opportunity we had at having one of the most beautiful earthly relationships. I look at the relationship my best friend Stuart has with his father and would have given anything to share that with you.

Movement IS Medicine

While it does not make it any easier to deal with, I do realize you had a disease called alcoholism. I knew it was real after one of your failed attempts at sobriety when you spoke to me and told me how your body "craved" the alcohol and that your body/mind experienced a euphoria and release when it was consumed. You said it was something only the alcohol could provide. I know this feeling. For me it is something only the love of Jesus provides for me.

Having this love in my heart allows me to honestly say two things to you. The first being I love you. While you have heard these words from me before, I have never said them as a married man with my own children. That is an important distinction for me because I now understand these words from a different perspective. A perspective that allows me to understand the impact and the void that our lack of a relationship created for us and ultimately creates for my children and me. But it is unconditional love that is at the foundation of my relationship with Christ. This is a love that I did absolutely nothing to earn. It's a love that is unconditional despite all of my flaws and imperfections. It's a love that I know is the greatest gift that I have ever received. And most of all, it's a love that requires me to give the same to you. The second thing this love allows me to say to you is that I forgive you. Those are words I have never written or spoken with the honesty and sincerity I do today. I am by no means perfect yet Christ looks past all of this and forgives me of my sin and transgression. Who would I be to receive this great gift from God and not offer you, my father, the same? There is a freeing and liberation that comes along with this. This is a liberation that will allow me to move on and have more effective relationships with my friends, family, wife, and most importantly my children.

I mentioned Grandma having two favorite hymns. The second was We Will Understand it better Bye and Bye. In closing, the third verse of this song says, "Trials dark on every hand, and we cannot understand all the ways that God would lead us to that promise land; but he guides us with his eye, and we will follow till we die, for we will understand it better by and by". As a child I never understood what this song meant, but as I have grown older it speaks magnitudes to my journey. While growing up fatherless may have been a dark moment in my life, I held on to God's unchanging hand and he delivered me out of this darkness. I have learned from this and am using this lesson to be a better friend, family member, father, and husband. I can testify to His goodness in delivering me out of this darkness and will follow him all the days of my life.

Love You,

WC Strader II

Weston C. Strader *is happily married and the proud father of a son and a daughter. While he has roots in the Philly suburbs, he and his family reside in Smithfield, VA where his kids attend a private Christian school and he and his wife hold positions within*

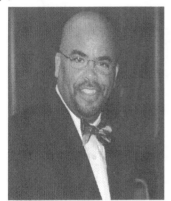

the finance and healthcare technology industries. Wes started his undergraduate studies at Millersville University but as life would lead him in many different directions, he completed his studies at Temple University where he was introduced to his beautiful bride. He is a proud member of Alpha Phi Alpha Fraternity. On the weekends he can be found cheering on his daughter's efforts on either the soccer field or basketball court and on Sunday morning can be found praising his Lord and Savior, Jesus Christ, at Harvest Fellowship Baptist church where he has been a member for over five years.

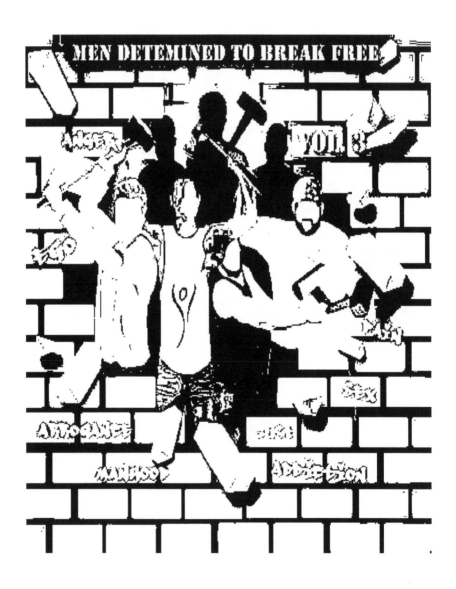

Chapter Three

Brown On the Outside A Person On the Inside
By
Aaron Dread

Breaking free is easy when you can identify your captors or the barriers that hold you back. But what happens when you can't identify your jailors, or measure the impact that their mental incarceration has had on your life? You stay lost or stuck in a rut until you can piece your life together and create your own identify and make a new path for yourself.

In Rev. Dr. Martin Luther King Jr's "I Have of Dream" speech, he envisioned, "...A world where a man would be judged not by the color of his skin but by the content of his character..." This seemingly simplistic expectation of life has been one of our greatest societal challenges. Unfortunately, racial discrimination and prejudice shows no signs of being diminished even in 2016. Human nature's fatal flaw of identifying and categorizing people by their skin color has left emotional, social, and financial scars on millions of individuals and on our society as a whole.

Like most boys that grew up in the late '70s or early '80s, we played outside all day long. We played football, basketball, and traded baseball cards from the time our parents went to work until the sun set. During one of these days, I was playing with a group of my friends in my neighborhood. The group consisted of two white brothers, their neighbor (who was an adopted black boy being raised by a white family) and myself. As normal with most pre-teen boys we played, we argued, and we fought. But this day was different. One of our normal arguments over a "call" in a football game ensued. I was arguing my point with the two white brothers and out of the nowhere the other black boy screamed out, "Shut up Nigger!" The environment that me and the other black boy were raised in had both of us trying to find our identities. Where did we belong? Who were we? How twisted was our environment where we would use such a hateful word that was frequently used by white people against each other.

I have spent a large part of my early years feeling very much like a square peg trying to fit into a round hole. Being raised as a mulatto child reared by my single white mother in ultra conservative Lancaster County created a series of identity issues that I was unaware that I even had until I reached my late 20's which I am still working through in my 40's. Society has very clearly defined social roles that create rigid boundaries between whites and blacks. The attitudes towards these roles have been my prison. I made a decision several years ago to finally break those shackles and embrace my own personal diversity. I am focused on being Brown on the outside and being the best person that I can on the inside. To the world I am clearly identifiable as a black man based on my skin color. The gift that I want to bring to the world is teaching others to embrace the diversity of thought, culture and personality, contrary to the racial stereotypes society has created for us.

The topic of race is always a controversial and sensitive topic. I always find it productive and credible to provide fair balance when discussing race. There are three areas of my life where I experienced significant events that created the mental imprisonment I've struggled with for years. The three areas where I have struggled with my racial identity and myself the most were: dating as a teen, through my college years, and within my professional career.

Dating may have been one of my more challenging experiences growing up. As the only black male in my graduating high school class of 400 plus students and one of ten blacks in the entire school, teenage dating was a difficult process. I recently talked to one of my dearest friends, a white female I have been a close friend with since the 3rd grade. She told me the first time I rode my bike over to her house in the fourth grade her Dad asked her what the neighbors would think. I had no less than three girls that I liked where their parents told the girls they were not allowed to date me because the color of my skin. I was a good student, popular among my group of friends and a star of the basketball team. In the face of this, the color of my skin was a limiting factor in dating. This began to have a significant impact on my self-confidence. In my sophomore year, my white mother sat me down and explained to me that I was not going to be accepted by the parents of these girls. She began taking me to events and encouraging me to go into Lancaster, a nearby city. I still remember her words to this day, " Go in Lancaster and find you a pretty brown girl." While I had much more success dating, I faced my ultimate dilemma, I didn't fit socially there either. I didn't listen to the same music, and I couldn't dance. I wasn't used to the urban lifestyle that they were a part of. I received probably more direct confrontation from other black kids because I didn't fit than I did from my white classmates in my school. This really sent me into a conundrum. I was really happy with who I was. It just felt like nobody else, whether they were white or black, was okay with where I fit in on the social spectrum. At this point in my development as a man, I was very unclear about where I belonged. I couldn't identify my oppressor. I didn't know whom to trust. This was the beginning of my mental captivity.

I was an accomplished high school basketball player. I believe I still hold the boy's high school scoring record at Penn Manor High School. My plan was to play college basketball while I pursued my degree. I had no idea what a culture shock college and playing collegiate basketball would be. My identity as a freshman in college was as a basketball player. In our social environment on the team, the black players primarily hung together. Most of my teammates were from Philadelphia or much more urban areas than Lancaster County. So I felt immense pressure to conform to their behaviors and attitudes. They made fun of my clothes, my haircuts and how I talked. It was a rough freshman year for my ego. The black women on campus also played an instrumental role in my evolution to self-worth as well. There was one. Those dang Girls High girls that had my naive country nose wide open. I really fell for her. However, her boyfriend in Philadelphia didn't seem to appreciate that fact. It would have been nice if I knew he existed. But this was just another valuable coming of age lesson. She was able to take advantage of my inexperience and my desire to fit in helped carry on her deceit. But it was ultimately a blessing in disguise. This was my first true exposure to the experience of a young black male in America. For the first time I had someone I played ball with, went to class with, ate three meals a day with and shared coming of age experiences with that looked like me. I began to change the way I dressed. My dialect changed. I drank and smoked for the first time. I felt so much pressure to fit in because I was harassed mercilessly for the way I talked and how I acted. They say when you apply pressure to a piece of coal; you end up with a diamond. I was under such social pressure to fit my peers' expectations that I began to develop and to adopt a self-worth and self-identity that I didn't possess before.

As I left college, ready to face the world, I thought I had found a comfort zone. I found a group that accepted me for who I was. I socially had allied myself with a black urban culture. I thought I had this all figured out until I met corporate America! I was thrust back into the tank I grew up in where I was in the minority. I was different again. In my first pharmaceutical job, I began to feel the pressure. When you come into a meeting or a dinner, do you sit with at a table where a few blacks have gathered or do you sit away from them to network with your white peers? I personally didn't care or have a preference. I fit in anywhere because of my ability to get along with others. However, I would receive sly comments from my black colleagues if I sat with the white group. Or one of my white colleagues would walk by the table where the blacks gathered and ask, "Is this the black table?" Simple things like this sent my psyche into a tailspin. I had been identified as a fast track employee targeted for placement in management in a few years. I was given classes on how to dress. I was assigned a personal coach to help me with my communication skills and how those perceived me I communicated with. They were creating the "me", that they wanted to create. I began to feel the person I had evolved into was slowly withering away. I was following the direction they were sending me and was continually being overlooked for promotions. I was provided feedback after interviews about my communication style. They often told me they were not sure if people would be able to handle my presence. After I began to analyze all the feedback I was getting, it all started to sound like, "You are too black. You are a tall, assertive, confident black male." However, that was exactly what I had been trying to become.

The various obstacles that I have shared were created by humans' desire to characterize by race or color of skin. This is a flaw in human nature, which leads to mental, emotional, and physical barriers that hold back our society and its members from reaching their full potential. Many very talented people spend way too much time trying to fit a stereotype to be accepted before they can let their true skills and value as a friend, mate, or employee shine through. My journey led me to a mental space where I learned to finally accept who I am. It also led to me to a place where I was able to minimize the value in other people's opinions of me. I no longer allow people to try to fit a square into a round hole just so they could put a label on me. I avoid narrow-minded brown people that practice this slave mentality. I smile in the face of white people that struggle to accept my intellect and talent because it does not fit into the role they have been taught about black males. To the naked eye, I clearly present as a black male. But this inherently is the problem! Black men, Caucasian men, Latino men, are not singular in thought, culture, or behavior. All humans are diverse in their makeup and should not be pigeonholed to fit into what the image society has created to for them. Categorizing and stereotyping people makes it easy for folks to identify them. A perfect example of this is the blatant racist rhetoric you see regarding President Barack Obama. The man is an intellectual giant. He has managed to get through two terms as a president without any moral or corruption scandals. While you may or may not agree with his politics, you would not be honest if you don't think much of the criticism and political rhetoric he receives is not largely due to his race not fitting the mental image of how people perceive the President of the United States. President Obama has brought the underlying racial opinions of many folks to the forefront. This concept of mental image and racial identity plays a huge role in the disconnect with President Obama being a square peg trying to fit in a round hole.

Brown on the outside, a person on the inside; this is a very simple concept. However, far too many people place more emphasis on the outside shell than the inside content.

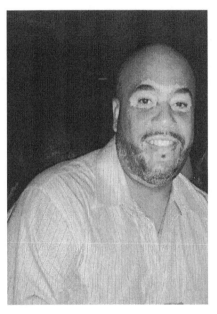

Aaron Dread is currently working as a sale professional in the pharmaceutical industry. His life experiences have led him to be happily married to Kisha Murray-Dread, and to be the father to 3 children, Myles 16, Malcolm 14, Mason 9. They currently reside in Burtonsville Maryland just a few minutes north of Washington DC. Aaron is actively involved in his fraternity Omega Psi Phi. He also is very involved in mentoring young men through AAU basketball in the Baltimore and Washington DC area.

Movement IS Medicine

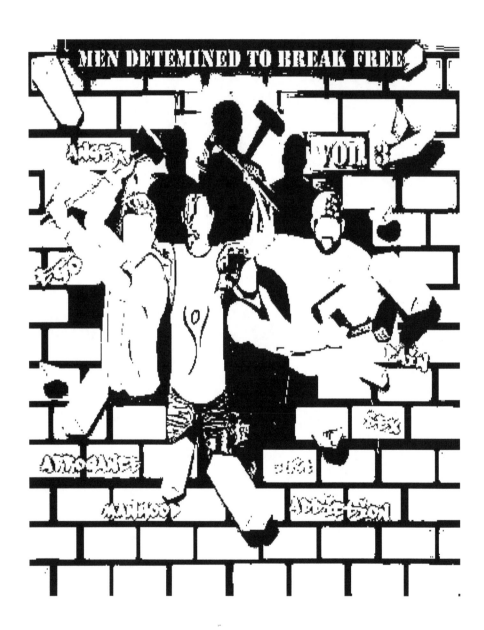

Chapter Four

My Life As It Is - Evening the S.C.O.R.E.
By
Jonathan Decoursey Edwards Jr.

I was around eight or nine years old when I became vaguely aware that I was different from most other people. At that time, I started to believe that I would probably have to deal with some major health complications or medical issues as an adult or my life might even be cut short early due to my health. Oddly enough, instead of being scared, sad or upset when I had these thoughts, I actually felt a slight feeling of delight rush through my mind as I would chuckle and think to myself, "Oh well, live fast, die young! I guess I'm gonna be outta here early, suckas!" These feelings surfaced one day after I was told that I had a disease called Sickle Cell Anemia by the nurses in my pediatrician's office. I remember I had asked why I had to get a needle that day. That's when they explained to me that Sickle Cell was a blood trait disease that I would have to live with for the rest of my life. I was told to make sure I always had a lot of water to drink in order to stay hydrated and they told me that if I ever felt any pains in my knees or other joints to make sure I told my parents or any adult at school because I could be experiencing a painful episode that people with Sickle Cell often suffer from which is known as a "crisis."

Fortunately for me as a child, I didn't suffer from pain crises or any major health dilemmas or the complications that many children with Sickle Cell endure like infections, organ damage and even strokes or any major surgeries. These ailments often cause people with the disease to constantly be in and out of the hospital. Occasionally, I would get fatigued riding my bike or playing outside or in school or get extra thirsty in the middle of class but for the most part, I was able to play basketball, race up and down my block and enjoy my childhood with my two younger sisters plus my cousins and friends.

Having Sickle Cell meant that I had to have my health monitored on a consistent basis. My mother would take me to Children's Hospital of Philadelphia monthly and the one thing that stood out to me at those visits was that there always seemed to be a lot of drama and chaos in the visitation room and even in the waiting room. There was loud crying and occasionally a shocking scream while a nurse would do her best to calm a highly upset child or wailing infant.

The nurse would say things like, "ok, you're going to feel a small pinch."

"Just look at me, don't look at it."

"It's going to happen really fast, ok?"

"If you sit still and stop crying, you can have this lollipop...don't you want a lollipop?"

You could hear this plea outside of the one particular room where they would draw blood and see kids come out with tear-soaked faces as well as, red-faced toddlers holding their elbows and sucking on a lollipop. I held my composure when it came to needles and was naturally very cool and calm. In all honesty, I was scared but it just wasn't in my nature to fall out screaming and crying like a crazy person when I was upset. My first grade teacher used to call me "Johnny Cool" due to my laid-back composure and the way I handled certain situations with relaxed coolness and nonchalance. Anyway, I took those needles during my hospital visit and they didn't really hurt at all. I received my colorful Snoopy Band-Aid and turned down the lollipop as my Mom and I walked back to the lobby to wait for the doctor to see us.

I enjoyed this special time with my mother because I got an excused day off from school and we would go downtown which was a whole new environment and experience. Plus, back then CHOP had a McDonalds in the lobby and you couldn't beat that as a kid. Wearing her work clothes and perfume, my mom seemed like a different person when we went to the hospital together. Sometimes she drove and sometimes we used the subway. It was fun and it was much better than a regular day at school. It was nice to get some alone time with my mother. I was the only boy in my family and the oldest child so my two younger sisters normally commanded most of my mother's attention. However, on those days when we went to visit my doctor for my Sickle Cell check-ups, it was a special time and I enjoyed undivided attention.

I had great parents who provided well for us. They weren't the helicopter parents that you see today and they weren't really passionate about anything except for making sure we got an education and kept a job. But every once and a while, they were encouraging about other things. One particular summer, they encouraged me to get the heck out of the house for the summer, even if it was only for a week and a half. CHOP was offering a chance for me to go to overnight camp for children with Sickle Cell. I thought to myself, "I don't want to go to that camp with all those sick kids. I'm not sickly like them! Plus, I don't even know any other kid with the disease. If I go, who am I going to play?" I was not happy. As an eleven-year-old, mentally and socially the whole idea seemed like a bad one for me. I just really did not want to be characterized as a sickly kid or lumped together with this bunch of kids that I didn't even know. I had a reputation to maintain. My mother assured me that everything was going to be fine as she claimed, "going away for a couple of weeks should be fun and any way, you're going, regardless of what you feel or think."

So, when we arrived at CHOP's parking lot for camp departure, I had my sleeping bag, Walkman and my Special Ed and Public Enemy cassette tapes (just in case I had to spend time on my own walking around kicking rocks or throwing stones onto the lake or something). We were about to board the bus and I was in a parking lot full of kids. Surprisingly, there were about 30-40 kids as well as, volunteer camp counselors who were college students and some young doctors who I had seen occasionally at the hospital. We were separated by age and stood around in our groups in front of the buses. My father was the type of outgoing, friendly guy who would start conversations with anyone who would give him a listening ear.

He started talking to a young lady and her son, Dwight. My parents introduced us and I looked at this kid who was a couple of inches shorter than me. I was surprised to find out that he was actually sixteen years old. He had a disfigured left arm from birth and he couldn't place his right foot all the way on the ground because he had a venous ulcer. It would cause pain if he applied any type of pressure from his body weight on his foot when he walked, so he kind of walked tippy-toed and off balance. Dwight was a very immature looking teenager. He and I hit it off pretty well and I kissed my parents good-bye.

Boarding the bus, I searched the aisles for a seat but all of them seemed to be taken by screaming children and camp counselors trying to settle in. I looked at one of the girls I saw in the parking lot earlier but another girl sat next to her. Then I looked to my left and there was Dwight, waving to me, "Hey John, sit here!" I agreed to sit with him only if he gave me the window seat and surprisingly, he let me have it. I thought to myself, "ok, my Walkman batteries are going to get worn out on this trip. I have nothing in common with this guy." I sat down and turned up the music and Dwight asked me what song I was listening to. "Night of the Living Baseheads," I responded. We talked a little bit about Public Enemy's latest album and I offered to let him listen to mines. I looked out the window as we left Philly heading on the highway. Both of us listened to music on our Walkman's as we drove to the camp. With many young guys, there is an unspoken code to building a friendship. We didn't just automatically start cracking jokes and talking non-stop but I was at ease with him and I remember thinking to myself that the trip might not be as bad as I thought it was going to be.

Arriving on the campgrounds, I took in all of the beautiful scenery and I noticed there was a lake for kayaking which was closed. The camp cabins including the walls and even bunk beds were made of a deep dark brown wood. We had tennis courts, a pool as well as, inside and outside basketball courts. In fact, the first argument that we had involved which court we would play on first as we argued over who could and couldn't dunk (in reality, I doubt that any of us could even reach the rim). We picked out our rooms and Dwight and I had bunk beds. There were six people all together in our cabin including two male college students named Dan and Eric and two other campers, Irving and Sean. Irving wanted to play for UNLV basketball team and he was from North Philly. He would constantly talk about both of these things but he was 13 years old, extremely short and had Sickle Cell Anemia but he was a good basketball player. Irving and the counselor Dan related to each other through the subject of basketball. Dan was a head counselor who had recently graduated medical school at either Penn or Drexel University. The thing that stood out to me about Dan was the fact that he was this tall white guy about 6 foot 4 inches with a thick red beard. Dan shared a room with Eric, our other head counselor. Eric had one more year to graduate from Haverford College and he looked like Adam Sandler with the same hairstyle. He actually was a pretty nice guy and they both asked us all of us a lot of questions. In fact, our entire cabin was a great crew when it came down to it.

Camp activities involved us playing basketball. Then we would go to the pool then scope out some of the cute girls. There was lunch then free time and after free time spent in our cabins, we usually slept or wandered the campgrounds. We met to talk about health with the doctors and counselors and then there was dinner. That was the basic schedule for the one week we were there. When it rained, we played on the inside courts. Honestly, to my surprise, I had a great time.

Two days before it was time to leave, we planned to prank the girls. Just like most overnight camps, there was always a huge competition between groups and the girls were pitted against the guys. There was a tug of war attack that started this rivalry earlier so the big pay back was coming. All of the boys got together, about twenty of us and under the direction of Eric and Dan and another counselor, we tied our t-shirts around our heads like ninjas, showing off our bird chests wearing basketball shorts. Some guys had flashlights as we crept around the camp at night under the moonlight. Breathing hard through our t-shirts, we all ran around taking our positions around the girls' cabin. We stood there under the steps of the cabin. The cabins were elevated off the ground by brick columns and you could walk in or hide under them if you were bold enough and not scared of spider webs or other ungodly woodland creatures that probably hid under there. So, we all had buckets of water balloons and some of us had water guns. This was before super soakers and I had a little handgun and a bigger water gun in the back of my shorts—in case I got captured. So the boys split into groups and we attacked the girls in their bunks. I made a point to target the vulnerable girls and the girls that I had a crush on. It was a great night, we had a blast! After a night of mayhem, we had plenty of talk and laughter about it the next morning.

Unfortunately, along with all young pre-teen fun and mischief, there was a "blah" ending. A kid got sick sleeping in a wet bed that night and had to go to the local hospital because he had a high temperature and actually went into a "crisis." A crisis is the sickling of the red blood cell, which clots your joints and causes severe pain for those with Sickle Cell. Crises are the most difficult condition that comes along with disease. So far, the only short-term cure for these episodes is painkillers and rehydrating the patient with intravenous fluids. The poor kid, I can imagine the pain he must have felt just from being in a water fight. So, we had two more days at camp and all the adults were handling our events with kid gloves.

The last night of camp, Dwight and I stayed up talking about his driving test and getting a car, going back to school and going back to Philly. I started thinking to myself that Dwight was five years older than me but looked and sounded younger than me. He was preparing to drive a car, go on his prom in another year and graduate from high school. I wasn't thinking that far down the line. He was going to achieve all these things but achieving them living with Sickle Cell Disease and I really didn't want anything to do with it. I wanted to be normal, a normal kid who could play basketball and football without getting tired five minutes in. I wanted to ride my bicycle all day and not worry about chance of a crisis and one who could sleep in a wet bed and not get extremely sick the next day. Even at the end of my camp experience, I kept thinking that I was just a "normal" red-blooded kid and Dwight's situation didn't apply to me. Little did I know Dwight and me had a lot more in common than I thought.

As I look back now, I can say that my camp experience was great in that I learned to be grateful for my situation and for my life and I enjoyed the time I spent with other children with Sickle Cell. As an adult who is with now a father and husband with many future aspirations, goals and dreams, I have come to grips with the fact that I must take care of myself, monitor my health and learn to live with Sickle Cell Disease.

In my early 20's, I was caught up in partying, clubbing, smoking cigarettes and abusing my body like I was invincible. I was young and simply determined to have as much fun as possible. All of that time that I disregarded the fact that I had Sickle Cell Disease, I ended acquired a leg ulcer on my right ankle that brought me face to face with the harsh realities of this disease. I had to go through three skin grafts and even got a stomach ulcer from taking too many Ibuprofen pain relievers. I finally can admit that this disease has taken a certain toll on my life in that it has taken away so much of my time and caused me a great deal of frustration constantly having to deal with the health care system. Furthermore, it took me a while to open up and tell others that I have Sickle Cell. I guess I just wanted to live a perfect life and l just wanted to be a perfect person even though l know now that there is no such thing.

So it turns out that the premonitions that I had of my life ending early due to Sickle Cell, merely gave me an excuse to live carefree and naïve. I automatically expected to have a short life span, which was merely the irrational thinking of an eight-year-old. At one time, people with the disease were not expected to live over 40 but I have just celebrated that birthday with my family and friends and I look forward to many more birthdays in the future. I have started my own charitable organization providing education and financial support for those with Sickle Cell Disease called SCORE (Sickle Cell Organization for Relief and Education). I thank God for the memories and experiences that I have been through and I hope my organization will bring more attention to this disease and to help others with Sickle Cell live an organic and happy life.

Jonathan Edwards Jr.

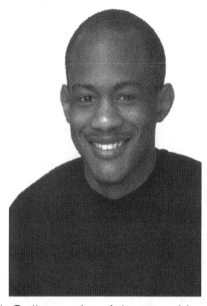

Jonathan D. Edwards, Jr. was born in Philadelphia and raised in the Mt. Airy section of the city. He is the oldest of three children born to Jonathan Edwards, Sr. and Carolyn Edwards. John grew up in and was confirmed at the historic St. Thomas African Episcopal Church and attended Saint Raymond's Catholic School, Leeds Middle School and Martin Luther King High School. Upon graduating from high school, John studied at Benedict College in South Carolina and Morris Brown College in Atlanta. He has a degree in Information Technology and has worked for more than ten years in the computer repair-helpdesk environment. He also has a certificate in computer forensics from Chestnut Hill College.

Jonathan is married to Adia Edwards and they have a 10-year-old son, Jacob Langston Edwards. At present, he is starting his own non-profit organization, SCORE that stands for Sickle Cell Organization for Relief and Education. His goal is to educate and to provide financial support to individuals inflicted with Sickle Cell Anemia.

John's hobbies include acting, traveling, playing his bass and acoustic guitars as well as, DJ-ing. His interests include writing and producing for film, theater and telev

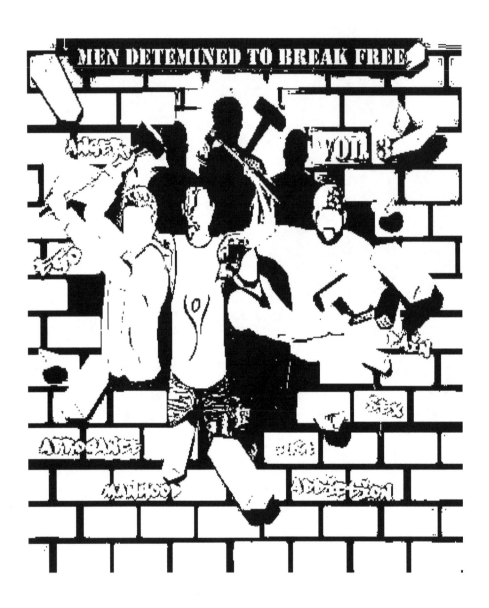

Chapter Five

Learning How to Survive: From a Young Man to Soldier
by
Robert A. McKnight

I was 14 years old when I was kicked out of the house. At first, I felt lonely and abandoned because it seemed like I didn't have anyone to turn to for help or support but I was also partly relieved. I was relieved because I didn't have to deal with any more drama with my Mom and the strict rules of our household, where I was secluded from interacting with the world. I moved in with the Mother of the neighborhood; we affectionately and respectfully called her "Mom" because she took care of everyone. If you didn't have a place to stay you, had a place at her house and food to eat. This was time in my life when I began to really get deep into the streets-stealing cars, robbing drug dealers, selling drugs and gambling. But the guys that I hung around with were like family and I was the youngest. They made sure I had a haircut, money in my pocket and they always made me go to school. I kind of enjoyed being in the streets because it was like a playground to me; I had no fear of anything. Any time I got into something, I had people there to back me up. I was locked up a few times due to my behavior in the streets.   It was never for anything major but still it was not the life I wanted to live.

The guys around me encouraged me to start dating girls. When I did I started going at them hard because that's all I saw my

Dad do; he had a different girl every day. I tried to be just like my Dad because I thought he was the coolest man in the world. Our relationship was shaky because there are always two sides to the story of why he wasn't around--I knew it was partly because my Mom didn't want him around and partly because he didn't know any better. Everybody raised him but his parents. He was always just so happy as long as he had a pocket full of money and a woman on his hip. My relationship with my Dad was more like homeboys or just friends than father and son. I did not really recognize or fully understand until years later on, that as a result of his upbringing, he gave me all that he could give. So I accepted what he was able to give. He was able to teach me how to be a good person to treat people the way you would want to be treated. As well as to always be a straight-up person and that would take me a long way in life. Even though he was uneducated, he also taught me about the importance of having and using common sense. He would always greet me with a, "Hey Sonny" and we would go from there. He had a personality that was bigger than life to me, which is why I looked up to him so much.

While still in high school I had way too much fun; I did what I wanted to when I wanted to do it. Eventually, I got kicked out of school in the eleventh grade so I started working full time. After about a year and half, I was encouraged by "Mom" to go back to high school and graduate. She was not someone you could say no to and get away with it. So, I decided to go back to high school to finish my education and to get things right so I could go to college. However, my pursuit of a college education was interrupted because I found out that I had a baby on the way. The happiest day of my life was when I found out that I had a son on the way. I said to myself, "I have to teach him the things that I did not get taught.

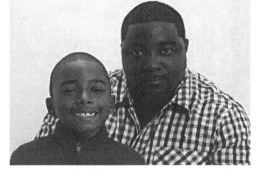

My son's mother wanted to go to college as well, so I decided to go to work full-time as a long shore man while she went to college. For the first couple of years, I spoiled my son. Then work slowed down on the waterfront so I had to come up with a new plan. I wanted my son to be proud of me and that is when I decided to go into the Marine Corp.

Joining the Marines was not all that it was cracked up to be. I did not know it was going to be that challenging. They definitely know how to bring you down and build you up into a machine. After about five months into the fleet, I was off to war. I was stationed in Al-Sad, Iraq. When I stepped off the plane it was like being in a movie, everything was in slow motion. I had to psych myself up as I thought, "I am here now." I could not allow fear to set in; it had to go out of the window. In my mind, I had to put on that suit of armor and get it done. While I was there I had no fear of anything, not even dying. Hearing the gunshots was just like being home. It was normal to hear them but ducking bullets every day and actually shooting people back every single day was different. There were just a lot of bombs going off around me. I was losing friends, brothers. I have been to Fallujah, Bagdad, Baghdadi, and Ramadi. I learned many lessons in the middle of war. One of the most important was that everyone has an emotional switch that they can switch on and switch off. We saw children that looked innocent, but we knew that they had bombs that could kill us in a matter of seconds if we let our emotions overrule us.

Although I have had to serve in the war, the military has afforded me the ability to travel and to see many distant lands. For example, I have been to Ireland, Germany, Kuwait as well as, other places stateside.

Coming back home after the war, I was in a lot of trouble. I didn't want to come back stateside to serve I wanted to stay in the war. I felt more comfortable over in the war than I felt state side. Over there I knew what to expect, coming home I did not. Here on home soil they will sneak you; you never know what people will do. Back in the States, I was an emotional wreck. I couldn't sleep; I was getting into arguments and fights. Overall, I was just an emotional mess. I received an "other than honorable discharge." I came home and found out I had Post-traumatic stress disorder known as PTSD and tendinitis in both knees. I was taken care of by the Veterans' Administration and then all of a sudden they cut me off. It took me three and half years and a lawyer for the VA to recognize me as a veteran and give me my benefits. I am now considered a disabled veteran that is unemployable. I struggle with the demons of war to this day seven years later.

My life will never be normal again as I know. It is what many call a "new normal." I can no longer stand loud noises, crowds of people, different attitudes and tight spaces.

Coming back home, many things have changed and some things have stayed the same. The one goal I had, which was to make my son proud of me and to be able to take care of him, I was able to achieve. The neighborhood Mom who encouraged me to finish my education passed away at the age of 96 and my dad eventually passed away as well. Before his passing I believe we were able to achieve the Father/son relationship that we were destined to have.

I hope my story helps others understand the many issues and setbacks that returning veterans face after fighting for their country. One will never know what it is to walk in my shoes.

Semper Fi

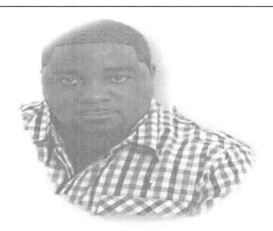

Robert A. McKnight is a native of Philadelphia Pennsylvania. He is eldest of his fraternal twin Runell A. McKnight by two minutes and one of seven siblings. Robert was an avid athlete through out his school years playing football and basketball. During his high school years Robert was apart of the MBA Business program for young future businesspersons. He traveled throughout the United States to various conferences with the program. Robert graduated from Regional High School in 2003. Shortly after high school Robert began working as a long shore man until 2006

In 2006 Robert enlisted in the united State Marine Corp Robert achieved the rank of Lance Corporal while participating in the Iraq War, Operation Iraqi Freedom. His job was title Task MP and was responsible for carrying out convoy security. Robert retuned home stateside from the Iraq War in 2009, and received an Honorable Discharge in 2013. Robert is the parent of one child, Semaj A. McKnight.

Movement IS Medicine

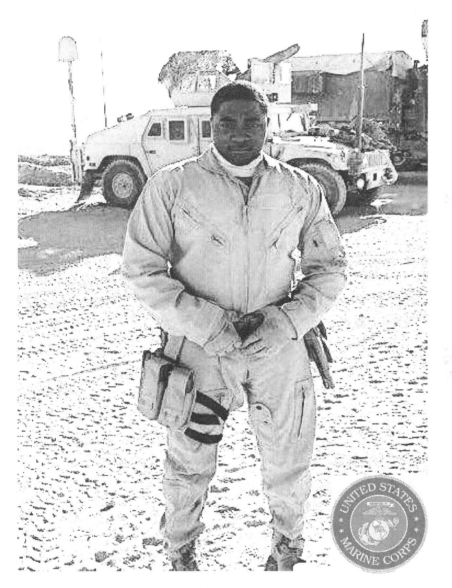

1982~2016
Rest well Marine Robert A. McKnight

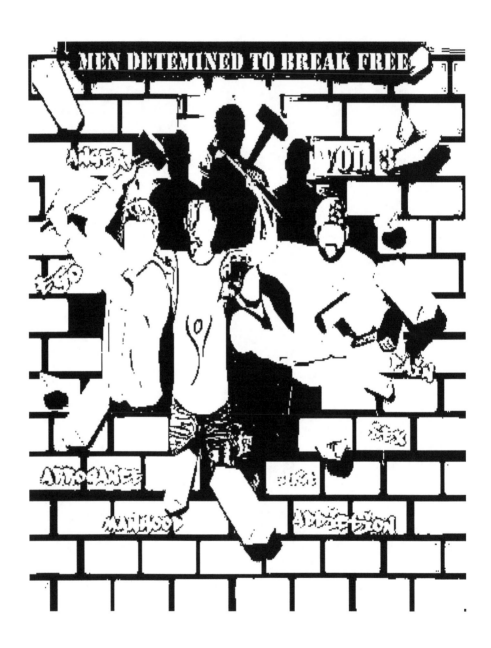

Chapter Six

A Warriors Song
By
Antonio D. Parker

Growing up in West Philadelphia and being raised by a single mother seemed normal to me. In fact, single mothers, primarily raised many of the kids in the neighborhood where I grew up. Although there were some kids who did have a father's presence in the home, many of my examples of manhood were provided by uncles and other men in the neighborhood. My father lived about two blocks over, in the projects on 46th street. Although I would see him on occasion, I've always known my father as man who people might view as being "crazy." I would see my father dressed in bummed out clothing, always carrying some sort of beat up books, unshaved, unkempt, un-groomed, and always touching things. And strangely, I received a lot attention when I walked through my father's neighborhood, with people exclaiming, "That Carlos' son!" "He looks just like him!" And in a weird kind of way, I relished the attention. I don't recall ever really being embarrassed by him or the way he looked or acted. I also was never angry towards him. I just accepted him for who he was. Whenever we would talk, he seemed to speak in his own cryptic language. And although I could grasp some of what he was trying to say, much of it went over my head. He would talk about the stars, mathematics, living on the 16th floor (in the projects) and more. Some of the things he would talk about seemed fascinating to me.

What probably made it easy for me to accept my father was because as different as he was, I too was a different. I have always been different. I never got caught up in materialism, or having name brand sneakers, or whatever the new fad was. I walked to the beat of my own drum. However, being different has not always been easy. Like any young kid growing up, I wanted to fit in and be accepted by my peers, and especially accepted by the girls. But I never seemed to possess that "It" factor. I've learned in life that some people just naturally have that quality that everyone seems to like and gravitate to, but I didn't seem to possess that quality. However, I have since learned that the secret to possessing that attractive quality is self-acceptance.

It took me many years to accept and love myself unconditionally. I had to learn to accept my dark skin, my thick lips, my short stature, and just being different. In an environment where European features were the standards of attractiveness, I seemed to be the antithesis—In fact; my features have strong African characteristics. And when I was coming up, few people, if any, in my circle of family and friends wanted to have anything to do with Africa, let alone look African. I didn't understand it at the time but the impact of racism, white supremacy and black self-hatred has had an insidious affect on the psyche of my community, and I always seemed to feel the brunt of that ignorance.

My journey has been particularly difficult because I didn't have many people in my life to validate me or reassure me that I was ok. Yet I have always displayed a positive, upbeat, and cheerful personality. I learned early in life how to smile through pain, laugh at myself and to build walls to protect myself. Life's curveballs have come at me in different ways: fatherlessness; rejection; heartbreak; racism; intra-racial self hatred; stereotypes; unfairness, to name a few.

Underneath my seemingly happy-go-lucky personality, was a militant spirit; I was a naturally born fighter. And whether I was fighting somebody around the block, or fighting life itself, I was determined to win life's challenges, and overcome any obstacle that came my way. Were it not for a deep internal drive, stubborn will, a pursuit of excellence, and God's divine will and favor, I might not have made it this far in my life.

I have always been more of a spiritual person. Although I went to Catholic schools early on in my life, and would often attend my grandmother's Baptist church, I have never have been much of a religious person. But those environments gave me my first concept of God and the idea of faith. Through my darkest moments I have had to rely on and communicate with God to help me through. There

81

were many times I even called myself getting mad at God. And even when it seemed like God didn't hear me, I somehow managed to keep moving forward.

Many of my life's challenges can be attributed to the impact of growing up in communities of dysfunction, living in a country that has oftentimes been hostile towards the African American community, and growing up in a community that has oftentimes been even more hostile towards itself.

Growing up in the Black community, having the "complexion of connection and affection" seemed to be only for those with lighter skin. Consequently, being the darkest of all my brothers, cousins and friends, I was able to see and experience the disadvantages of having dark skin, while witnessing the advantages afforded to those lighter-skinned folks. Witnessed this intra-racial phenomenon long before I became aware of the inequities in the group dynamic between Black and White people.

No one really knew the deep emotional pain I endured because I didn't look a certain way, act a certain way, or because I was different. Most people would look at-my happy go lucky external façade, and make whatever assumption about me based on that. But what lurked beneath that smiling face, crazy and energetic personality, and even that flair of overconfidence was a person looking to feel loved accepted and validated.

Despite the rejection that I have experienced, it was a fierce determination and belief in myself that helped me to persevere. God also blessed me with the gift of music at the young age of ten. It was this passion for music that drove me. When I played my saxophone, I receive attention, encouragement and support from my community; as well as my peers. I was doing something that nobody in the neighborhood or within my family was doing.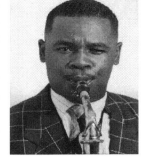

Movement IS Medicine

When I found music, I found my calling. It was the one constant in my life. If it wasn't for music, I don't know where I would be or how I would have turned out. Not only did playing the saxophone make me feel special, it also gave me direction and focus. It taught me discipline and gave me purpose. It gave me a dream.

The path towards musical excellence has taken me from playing on the street corners of downtown Philadelphia, to performing in different parts of the world. I can say literally that I went from "the streets to the suites," having performed in front of various U.S. Presidents, Congressmen, Diplomats and other dignitaries. I was also selected as a USIA Jazz Ambassador to seven countries in Africa, including Nigeria, Ghana, Togo, Zaire, Congo, Morocco, and Tunisia. I have performed in front of the Pyramids in Egypt. Additionally, I performed in different countries in Europe, and in Japan. I have been blessed to perform and record with many wonderful musicians and well-known artists. I have also been a music educator for almost twenty years. Moreover, because I continue to follow my passions, I continue to envision great things happening in the future.

Today, I can say that I'm a warrior and survivor. I'm a warrior because I never stopped fighting and believing in myself. I've learned (and continuing to learn) how to love and accept myself as God made me. And though even today I can look in the mirror and see the scars of my past, I'm still smiling. I'm still standing. I'm still striving to reach greater heights. I'm a survivor because America wanted me to fail; to become a statistic and to see myself as a victim. However, if I died today, I could proudly say that I've made a difference in peoples' lives. I can say that I have learned the true meaning of fatherhood; as I've been there for my own children since they were born. I can say I helped to make America better by educating young minds and exposing them to the art of music. Lastly, I can say that I shared my gift of music with the world.

My life's experiences could take up a whole book. But it was what a Howard University professor said to me that have helped me to put my life, and life in general, in perspective. He said, "All men are not created equal!" That statement had an impact on me. It changed my paradigm. It helped me to accept life for what it is. It helped me to see that the world is no utopian place. And as the great motivational speaker, Les Brown would say, "Life is a fight for territory. And the minute you stop fighting for what you want, what you don't want will automatically take over." After considering these wise words, I stopped looking for things to be fair and instead began focusing on my unique advantages. I began to appreciate my unique blessings. An unfortunate truth is that in life, even God's favor doesn't seem fair. So anytime I'm faced with some personal challenges, setbacks or disappointments, I tell myself that somewhere in the world there's someone who would gladly accept the "problems" that I have. It's all about perspective.

Finally, at this point in my life, it's about legacy. I want to suck the opportunity out of every second of living. I want to live a life of meaning and fulfilled purpose. I want to contribute something that will outlive me and in so doing, I want to help make the world a better place.

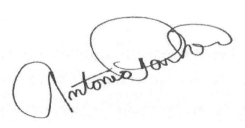

Movement IS Medicine

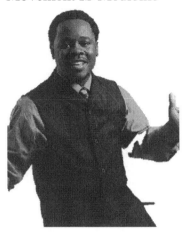

*Saxophonist, composer, educator and music songwriter/producer, **Antonio Parker**, is a native of Philadelphia, Pa. He is well known for his dynamic, energetic, and virtuosic performances as well as his versatility in a variety of musical styles. His artistry is deeply rooted in the jazz tradition but incorporates a wide spectrum of musical influences. He is a visionary artist who has been performing nationally and internationally for over 20 years. Antonio began playing the saxophone at the age of 10 and would later begin taking private saxophone and piano lessons at the Settlement Music School in Philadelphia. It was at Settlement, where Antonio would be exposed to the sounds and rhythms of jazz music. He would also be exposed to the music of the great alto saxophonist, Charlie Parker. In an instance, jazz would become the focus of his musical pursuits. At Settlement, Antonio was part of the jazz sextet and also performed in The Settlement Summer Music Program. It was through these programs that Antonio would meet other young, talented musicians throughout the city. He, along with renowned jazz bassist Christian McBride, and pianist/organist Joey Defrancesco were a part of The Philadelphia All- City Jazz Band during their high school years. They also attended the Philadelphia High School for the Creative and Performing Arts (CAPA). During high school, Antonio was the recipient of several scholarship awards, including, the Count Basie*

Scholarship, The McCoy Tyner Scholarship and was also awarded a brand new Selmer Saxophone. After graduating high school, Antonio entered Howard University in Washington DC, where he was given several special-talent scholarships to attend. He was a part of the Howard University Jazz Ensemble, where he has written, recorded and toured with the band. He has been a fixture in the Washington DC Metropolitan Area every since. Antonio's artistic achievements are many, and include serving as a USIA (United States Information Agency) Jazz Ambassador to 7 countries in Africa, where he performed and conducted jazz workshops in Nigeria, Ghana, Togo, Zaire, Congo, Morocco, and Tunisia. He has toured and performed in countries such as Japan, London, Scotland, Paris, Spain, Canada and Austria. He has also performed at the pyramids in Egypt with Smithsonian Jazz Masterworks Orchestra. Antonio has recorded and/or shared the stage with many well-known artists and entertainers, including Go-Go legend Chuck Brown, The Blackbyrds, The Ojays, Peabo Bryson, Ruben Studdard, Betty Carter, Illinois Jaquet, Jean Carne, Christian Mcbride, and many others. His debut CD, entitled "The Exchange" was well received and as was his follow-up recording, "Steppin' Out: Live @ HR57." His latest recording, "Planetentiary" fuses the sounds of jazz, funk and fusion, is scheduled to be released on his Airegin Label in early 2016.

Antonio is a graduate of Howard University, where he received his Bachelor of Music in Jazz Studies and his Masters degree in Composition & Arranging. He acquired a second Bachelors degree in Music Education from the University of the District of Columbia as well. As an educator, Antonio has taught in the District of Columbia Public Schools as well as Prince George's County Public School system. He is the founder and executive director of the Inner City Jazz Foundation and continues to educate young people on the importance of jazz music. His company, Mr. Parker Music Teacher, LLC focuses on creating and providing educational products and services to school-age children through the medium of music. In early 2016 Antonio will release a 17 book series entitled, "The Language of Jazz: A Repository of Melodic Ideas and Linear Constructions" through his latest company Jazzology publications, LLC.

Movement IS Medicine

~The Bridge~

Queen (I ain't mad at you)

The dictionary defines you as a woman who is foremost or
preeminent in any respect...
Prominent, distinguished and noteworthy.
Queen, I apologize...this is your King speaking.

I apologize for the times I've failed to treat you as such by
definition.
Recognition, sometimes blinded by remnants of our oppressive
condition.
The breakdown of my submission to the King of Kings gave rise
to the breakdown of your submission to me...
and I still see, Willie Lynch letter laced traces in your so-called
"Black Woman Attitude".
But to my God in heaven for you I still show gratitude,
graciously.
And I ain't mad at you, although I used to be!
See God's been working on me so I can better learn how to pray
for thee,
I just hope thee will do likewise for me.

I found myself at times being jealous of your climb up the
corporate ladder of success
not realizing it was designed for you to rise higher than your
King.
The bling from your shine should have made me want to support
and uplift
but instead I felt blind.
Yet when you mind your business more so than your King
succumbing to this conquering can emanate from a great divide.
Injury gets seasoned with insult, cooking up this recipe for
resentment as feelings of disrespect as uselessness sting my pride.
Emasculation, all be it like a tide washes away sense of purpose
and what's worse this ability you once had to properly define
feminine strength.
Look I know there's an account with which you can come up for
every time you feel I've failed to step up.

But if you try step into my shoes in lieu cause you think I've
refused then woman we both lose!
Not Queens but fools choose the views of a Godless society,
confused.
Cause they don't love or respect the rules.
Nor do they thirst for the water living in Proverbs 31 about the
virtuous one, worth much more than jewels. She is worth much more
than jewels!
But I ain't mad at you, although I used to be.
See God's been working on me so I can better learn how to pray
for thee.
I just hope thee will do likewise for me. The aftermath of the
diaspora ensues a plethora of issues
like mommas trying to fill daddy's shoes.
Mo' blues, that ain't never been mo' betta'.
Just bleak like Gilliam, yet mo' bitter than sweet sin to them who
let the trials of a fatherless life devise vices that divide a people, in a
world so cold and lifeless!
When all along these trials belong at the foot of the cross, where
Christ is.

I hear you crying out Sis,
and I know you need an escape from this crisis but you don't
understand,
as a temple your body's priceless!
Man I get stressed when I find you trying to find yourself while
losing your mind,
and half your clothes as you expose to the entire world what was
meant for only
one man to behold!
Displayed and sold like auction block livestock to the highest
bidder
striking a deal over your package.
Psychological damage from a sex cycle so vicious.

Movement IS Medicine

Psyched out and recycled through so-called men who stake
claims with their love lies fictitious.
It's insane, I mean ridiculous, the way your flesh has always been
on their wish list!
And ohh how I wish this insidious behavior so malicious and
malign would succumb to the divine enlightenment of the Savior
"Lord save her from these spineless swine!"
Cause you savor those mind altering lines they whisper in your
ear to get you so lifted as if to be suspended in time, uncontrolled,
casting your pearls at every fork in the road...
Like you're blind and can't read the signs.
You've been spent, as I lament, cause you were meant to be
bought with a price by Christ, from the Father, heaven sent.
But I ain't mad at you, although I used to be.
See God's been working on me so I could better learn how to
pray for thee.
I just hope thee will do likewise for me.

By
Thomas "Tiz" Fitzhugh

~Crossing Over~

Movement IS Medicine

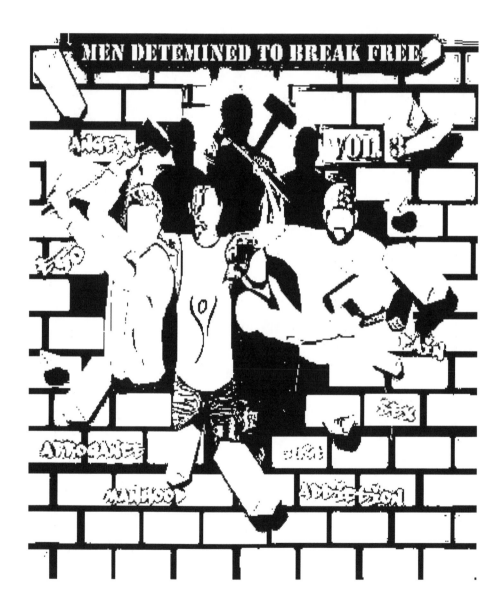

Chapter Seven

The Danger of Self-Disqualification
By
Rakeem S. Thomas

And do not be conformed to this world [any longer with its superficial values and customs], but be [a] transformed and progressively changed [as you mature spiritually] by the renewing of your mind [focusing on godly values and ethical attitudes], so that you may prove [for yourselves] what the will of God is, that which is good and acceptable and perfect [in His plan and purpose for you].

-Romans 12:2 (AMP)

We live in a culture where we put our security in the wrong things. We put our security in our abilities, our accomplishments, and our thoughts. When we put our security in ourselves, we determine if we have the ability to do something or not. Sometimes we put our security in people. We allow them to determine what we can and cannot do. These are all blockages that prevent us from living to our fullest potential. We begin to measure our lives and our abilities to our small minds and/ or the minds of others. It will lead to insecurity that will lead to self-disqualification.

If you're anything like me, then the word 'disqualify' is a close companion of yours. For the record, I am a rule follower. Always have been. Someone says something about the way I should live, or what can and can't be done during a certain season of life, and you know what, I'm all ears. Now, don't get me wrong, I'm not a push over (except when it comes to sweets... but I digress.) I definitely have a strong sense of who I am, and who God has called me to be, but I must admit I have experienced and have had encounters with this ugly undertone of self-disqualification in my life.

As far back as I can remember, I have always been my worst

critic. As I reflect over the years, I found myself battling the demon of insecurity. I thought I was ugly. I thought I was a nerd. I thought I would never get far in life. I thought it was meant for me to struggle all my life. Yes, I had dreams, goals, and aspirations. However, I was always downgrading myself, which would lead to disqualifying myself from the destiny God had for me.

Growing up was a struggle. I was a product of a broken home. My parents divorced during my early teenage years. From second to ninth grade, I was labeled a 'behavioral liability' in school; therefore placed in Behavioral Management, a.k.a. Special Ed. classes. I wasn't even allowed to ride on the same bus as the 'normal kids'. How embarrassing that was. Having to live with my grandparents for some time and other relatives, I felt abandoned by my parents. I never really connected with my biological father, I was separated from my siblings, and I lived in a home where I witnessed consistent child and parent domestic violence (a child physically harming their parent). During one horrific experience, I had a gun put to my head by an uncle who hated me. I was even rejected by 'church folk'. All of these things happened to me and I had no control over it.

As I got older, I was kicked out at 18. Fortunately, my father took me in. I found refuge in a relationship that I just knew was going to be my 'forever'. I was in love (so I thought). Five years of investing love, devotion, time, and even money, then my dreams of marrying her crumbled when she cheated on me. I was damaged, distraught, and discouraged. I give up on love and relationships completely.

The struggle was real and raw. While dealing with all of this in my younger years, I began to develop bouts of depression, suicide, and insecurity. I had lost hope. I began to feel like I had no worth to anybody or myself. I wanted to throw in towel. I began to settle. I began to allow all of the negative emotions to become the author of my destiny. I looked at my reality and began to disqualify myself from the very things God had in store for my life.

What I didn't realize was, I was in a war. I was in a war with myself, the war of self-disqualification. I was guilty of disqualifying myself from the things God had for me. I was guilty of hindering my own opportunities. While many people talk about their 'haters', I was my own hater. When I explored below the surface of many situations I experienced, I repeatedly found that my greatest barrier to growth, expansion, and taking positive action was...ME! I was wasting time. I was focusing on the wrong things. I was withering away due to self-disqualification.

I would disqualify myself from different aspects of life: "Oh, I can't do public speaking"; what if I stutter, or what if they laugh at me, or what if I forget the words I intended to say. Oh, I couldn't possibly go out of my way to introduce myself to a beautiful female, even if she is showing signs of interest. I want to get to know her... what if she isn't as interested in me, as I am in her. Oh, I couldn't fulfill my dream of making six figures, I have no college degree, and I don't even know if I had anyone in my family that made six figures. All I'm good for is flipping burgers at Burger King and maybe one day I'll be the manager and that's when the big bucks (30-40,000) will come. Oh, I can't preach. I feel it in me, I feel led, but my pastor won't even acknowledge the calling on my life. I guess God told him I wasn't called to preach. You can't pastor a church, I can't be a father, and I'm not good enough to be a husband". And on and on it goes...I was getting tired of allowing my insecurities to keep me from the victories God had in store for my life. I decided to start ignoring all of the excuses, and dare I say...lies, about what I could or could not do, what I'm qualified to do, and what I don't feel qualified to do, whatsoever. I began to look at my "I can'ts" and began to replace them with the question "why not?" When I began to courageously look at my excuses, the determination to see "what if" began to kick in.

What if... what if I decided to re-qualify myself for the life I've always hoped for? What if I actually believed that I had been created to be a blessing to others? What if I would stop being so insecure with myself? What if I could beat the odds in my family and be a breaker of generational curses? What if I could see myself as better than I have been? What would happen?

Within ourselves lie our best selves. We are created and designed to be something great. We are created with such great potential, that our lives are brimming with possibility. We have to take a really good look, re-qualify ourselves and keep exploring; why were we created, who we are, what our purpose in life is, and what we can contribute to others.

The Apostle Paul, wrote in the letter to the Galatians: "Make a careful exploration of who you are and the work you have been given, and then sink yourself into that. Don't be impressed with yourself. Don't compare yourself with others. Each of you must take responsibility for doing the creative best you can with your own life." (Galatians 6:4-5 MSG). Meaning, you cannot be trapped by the capacity of your thoughts and the thoughts of others concerning you. When you find yourself downplaying your abilities to achieve, gain, or succeed, you have to look beyond your perception and discover your purpose. You were created for an awesome purpose. When you focus on your purpose, you will progress in anything set before you. This is a fight. It's you verses you. You cannot afford to allow yourself to be defeated by you. You have to be determined to not allow self-disqualification to steal your inner potential. If you allow self-disqualification to steal your inner potential, it will keep you from your outward purpose in life.

The objective in overcoming self-disqualification is to take hold of the possibility and potential that God has placed in each one of us, and take the risk to re-qualify ourselves for the things we had always hoped we could do, but never believed we'd be able to. It's taking yourself back from the forces that are pushing you away from who you are destined to be. Don't delay or deny yourself from the purposes, plans, and places that God has already deemed you qualified for. Kill the noise of fear and turn up the volume of faith.

A lot of times God blesses us with opportunities not to work for, but to work in. In other words, God gives you opportunities for you to express & exhibit your gift. The sad reality is that some of us aren't doing much with our gifts because we keep disqualifying ourselves and robbing any potential within, hence we're missing out on opportunities that our lives present us because our gifts are unemployed. The enemy does not want you to enter into the abundance God has for your life. He will use the weaknesses on the inside of you and to try to overpower the favor that's on you. Every time I would try to do something I felt was for me to do, I would shy away from it because I was insecure. My insecurity would ultimately disqualify me from doing something that was really meant for me to do. What better way than to get you to disqualify yourself from what you are destined to receive.

If we're not careful we will allow our insecurities and issues talk us out of our blessings. I don't even want to begin to think about how many blessings I missed out on due to self-disqualification. We find lots of ways to disqualify ourselves: we don't have enough training or experience; we could never do it as well as someone else we admire; we are too something- young, old, fat, thin, shy, sensitive, inarticulate, etc. Meanwhile what God has for you can't be for you because YOU ARE IN THE WAY!

What would you do, if you knew you were qualified to live the life you've always wanted? The gifts of God are eternal. They are before repentance. Yes, that's what the Bible says. Ever wonder why there are so many talented people out there? That's how God made them. And He is so good that He gives us all gifts and He doesn't take them back either.

Being perfect is not based on what we do. It is not to be without fault. We all have faults. We all have shortcomings. The Bible definition of perfect is to be complete – and in Christ we are. All of our weaknesses He uses to display His glory and His strength. We are whole, we are complete, and we are finished in Christ. Just be.

Repent of disqualifying yourself. Don't allow bad reports to put you in a state of discouragement, and throw in the towel. It's easier to quit than to take a stand and say, "No, I will not fail. I do not receive that, in Jesus Name." God doesn't make junk. You have to stop criticizing yourself because when you do, you are criticizing something God had made. Who are we to criticize Him and His handiwork?

So…how do we step beyond all the limits we place on ourselves and begin living as though we are all sparks of something great?

Notice your unique style of disqualifying yourself

Sometimes we hold ourselves back in very subtle ways and it is up to us to sort out and begin shifting those old habits. Pay attention to the stories you are thinking in your head when faced with a challenging situation. Write down every time you speak in absolutes like 'never' and 'always' that lock you into one way of being. Notice how you judge yourself in comparison to others you admire. The goal is for you to unpack and rewire those habitual thought patterns and fears.

Accept praise graciously

All too often we brush aside or discount positive feedback from others. Many times we think playing down a compliment is being humble. It's actually showing insecurities. Every time you receive a compliment, place your hand over your heart center, take in the positive intent, and let the person know that it feels good to be appreciated.

Celebrate little successes

It may be hard to trust your personal qualities and power because successes pass by with little fanfare. Start doing nice things for yourself. Take yourself out to dinner. Treat yourself to the spa. Exercise. These things are simple, but they can go a long way if you make it part of your annual routine. Always remember, YOU ARE WORTH IT

Establish a new practice of s-t-r-e-t-c-h-ing your comfort zone

Begin by making a list of areas in your life that feel stagnant, frustrating, or stuck. Next, brainstorm (alone or with a trusted friend) 5-10 very specific action items under each area- with no editing for how "do-able" or scary that action seems. Pick one action item a week to try. Remember that this is not an exercise in how to do everything "right" or "perfect." Some will work and some won't, but taking the actions begins to train you not to stop at your traditional edge of comfort.

As a man in my 30's, I'd love to tell you how I have it all figured out. Honestly, I haven't. I have learned to tell myself that if you suck, you're human. Even that mantra doesn't always ease the pain. Risking failure is hard, irrationally hard. However, there is too much at stake to allow self-disqualification to abort the intent of God for our lives. When God becomes your joy, self-disqualification loses value in your life.

I reflect over my life and remember countless times when I disqualified myself. I cannot imagine where I would be today if I didn't have the determination and the drive to push through the walls of self-disqualification. I don't know how far I would have gotten if I had not shut the door on negative people and forces, surrounded myself with positive people who influenced me, encouraged me, empowered me through words and deeds. I would've never pursued my call to preach. I would've never left Burger King to eventually become a top car salesman. I would've never made my first six-figure salary at the age of 23. I would've never been married…with children. I would've never become the pastor of a prominent and progressive church. I would've never been a contributing author of this book. My story and my testimony would have never been heard. As a result, other's lives may have never been impacted. There would have been a whole lot of "never's" that would have led me nowhere.

Always know that you can overcome any obstacle life throws your way. Challenges are inevitable. However, defeat is optional. Be determined that the rest of your life will be the best of your life. Be determined to move in the direction of days popping and shining, bursting and expanding in you for life. Be determined not to give into the notion that all of life is really all we know. Instead, be a person who finds him or her self trying new things, exploring themselves and their world in a deep way, so that they end up living deeply creative, whimsical, and fully committed lives for a tremendous cause. Move forward persevering. Move forward determined. Move forward knowing you are qualified by God.

Move because you matter and your life is a gift designed to make a difference. Never disqualify yourself or count yourself out. As long as you never give up you will always have a chance. I did and I am glad to say, thank God, I'm well on my way!

Bye Self-Disqualification. Hi Self-Determination.

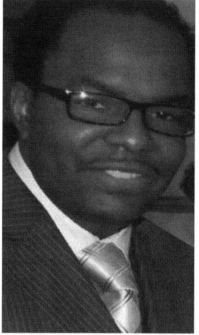

Rakeem Thomas is a follower of Jesus, husband, father, pastor, speaker, contributing author, visionary, and leader. He is the Senior Servant/Pastor of Mount Pleasant Church in Newark, NJ. Under Pastor Rakeem's leadership; Mount Pleasant has been tremendously blessed in areas of worship, membership, discipleship, stewardship, and leadership. He has led this congregation faithfully for over the past 5 years.

In addition to his role as a visionary leader, Pastor Rakeem has been blessed with the unique ability to connect with individuals on a personal and spiritual level. One of Pastor Rakeem's greatest passions is to effectively present the same relevant message-the good news of Jesus Christ- using fresh and innovative methods. Pastor Rakeem is a well sought after speaker/preacher/teacher/ revivalist/ leadership coach and has had the privilege to share his ministry throughout the country.

Pastor Rakeem's educational experience includes studies and majors in Pastoral Studies from Cairn University and New York Theological Seminary.

Pastor Rakeem and his wife, Jocelyn have two gifted children-Savannah and Rakeem Jr.

Pastor Rakeem's life scriptures are Psalms 1 and Matthew 6:33

Movement IS Medicine

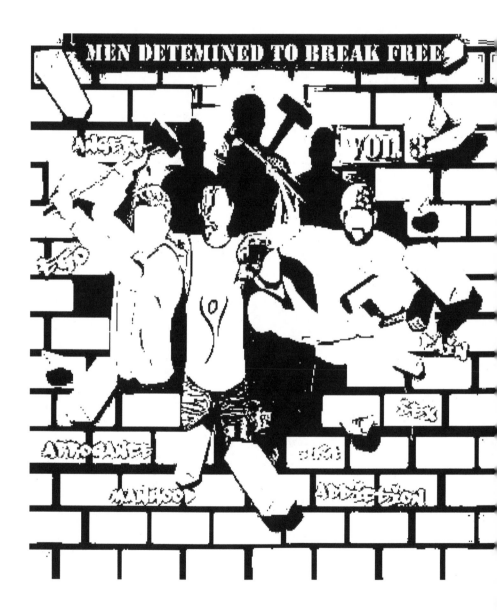

Chapter Eight

Redefining Profit

"Find your passion and your profit will follow"

By

Fred Waller EA, CFP@

In order to find success, whether it be in business, family life or some other aspect of living, there is one thing that I have learned:
With purpose comes profit. Follow your purpose and the profit will come.
Bishop T.D. Jakes

A few days after Ramona asked me to participate in this project, a couple of things happened that really helped me to form my thoughts. There was a Facebook video going around with Steve Harvey talking about "Jumping." If you haven't seen it, stop reading this and Google search "Steve Harvey Jump Video." He was finishing up taping Family Feud and was talking to the studio audience. He told a really motivational story about jumping. He said that "You can't just exist in this life, you have to jump." That really helped to put in perspective, for me, a unique moment in my life. Within a day or two of hearing that, I heard something else very powerful. When I'm at my office doing tax returns, I look for YouTube videos from T.D. Jakes, Keith Battle, or maybe a Ted Talk to play in the background while I'm working. On that day, I listened to a sermon from Bishop T. D. Jakes. In that sermon, he made that quote I referenced above. He said, "Follow your purpose." Notice he said, follow YOUR purpose. Nobody has a problem wanting to know his or her purpose in life. Some even take the steps to SEEK out their purpose, but something really, really powerful happens when you FOLLOW your purpose. I did that, and wow......

A little over 10 years ago, I was teaching middle school mathematics within the School District of Lancaster, Pennsylvania. It was a job that brought me joy and satisfaction; I enjoy teaching very much and I was happy to serve my students.

Seeing students gain mathematical concepts while developing as leaders brought me a lot of gratification for a long time. However, after about my fourth year, I started to desire something different. I began to get the entrepreneurial bug that developed into another passion.

At the same time that this new passion was rising within me, I noticed that I was beginning to want more out of life in general. I needed to find a greater level of success and happiness in my work that spoke to the purpose for my life. When starting to seek my purpose, I would often sit in meetings with teachers who had been educators for more than twenty years. And although I had only three to four years in, I was becoming disillusioned by what I saw. I still had the youthful zeal of a new teacher and wanted to implement new, refreshing ways of educating our children. But the teachers with whom I worked—were often jaded and bitter. They seemed to have been hardened by years of routine that held no level of success. More than anything, I did not want to work in a field where I would end up hating my vocation, and becoming mean and numb to the work of my hands.

In addition to becoming frustrated watching my co-workers basically becoming really negative, I was also getting frustrated watching students who didn't bring any level of energy to their education. I was beginning to feel like I was more invested in my students then they were in themselves. This led to a lot of discouragement on my part, and increased my desire to leave. It also increased my desire to work in a field where I could effectively motivate people and serve them with joy.

While seeing this and feeling this way, I was also realizing that at home, I wanted to be more available for my two little girls. My wife is also in education (a school administrator) and her job demands were increasing at the time. I thought that it would be great if one of us had a flexible work schedule that lent itself to being more accessible to the children and family. I wanted to be available to my own children more while also doing something that would allow me to scratch that entrepreneurial itch.

So, around 1999, I took a course to learn how to do taxes for people. I did that because my mother-in-law did taxes, and she told me that during tax season she never had to cash her checks from her main job. I then was starting doing taxes out of my home, that first year with about 14 clients. Over the next 7 years, I would work as a teacher full time and do taxes at home in the evenings. I didn't move right away. When I left, I was making about $55,000 a year as a teacher. At that same time, I was maybe making around $7,000 doing taxes for people. For whatever reason, I felt like I had to follow my purpose. Now, to be clear, my purpose at the time wasn't to make money. It was to actually help to create a healthy family atmosphere. Clearly, I wasn't following profit. I was following what I thought was my purpose as a husband and father, but what happened next, blew my mind.

Because I am a person of faith, after making the jump to a job that I felt more purposeful in, I would later realize that God wanted me in a career where the fruit of relationship building and impacting people could be seen. This was not the primary motivation for me in changing career paths, but an added benefit. I believe that while I was yearning to build a better life for my family, and me, God was urging me to encourage and serve others. This was how I came to live out His purpose for me on earth. I believe that if there is a strong thread that can come out of my story, it is that God desires us to have a strong purpose and meaning to our lives, both, for the benefit of ourselves and that of others. Major moves are sometimes how to get to those places.

So, I made the transition from a salaried educator in the public school system to an entrepreneur, doing taxes and eventually, becoming a Certified Financial Planner ™. I truly believe that you have to take leaps of faith when you desire to transition into a new life. Those leaps are often times uncomfortable and scary, but they are necessary to the process. As I began my transition away from a formal teaching career to one in the financial services industry, I had to trust that the uncomfortable feelings that I sometimes felt in the process were going to lead to a greater sense of purpose and prosperity.

After deciding to follow what I believed to be my purpose as a father and husband, and become a business owner with a flexible schedule, I very quickly found that being a trained educator gave me an advantage in my new field. I was able to teach people about other things like budgeting, financial management and creative motivation, while I was doing their taxes. The very place I had come from (education) was now equipping and helping me to be better at fulfilling my passion in life.

There were many hurdles and obstacles that I had to overcome in order to build my business. Living in Central Pennsylvania and being one of the only tax preparers and financial advisors of color; discrimination played a part in my journey. I found that many times I had to be almost perfect in order to convince people that I was worthy of their business. I also found that unfortunately, I was overcoming prejudice on two sides. I was working in a predominantly Caucasian area, but could not rely on people of color to utilize my business. I also had to work at maintaining pricing and standards that kept my doors open. This does not mean that I do not serve people of color, nor does it mean that they are the only ones looking to pay less for my professional services. It simply means that I had to learn to maintain professional business standards regardless of a client's ethnicity. I learned that if I wanted to be around long term in order to help all people, I needed to maintain equal pricing and practices.

In spite of these hurdles, I am happy to say that I have a mentality that places-high value on my own abilities. This helped me immensely when I realized that mentorship and help from others in building my business was not going to be available to me. The financial services industry is competitive; people don't often want to mentor you because they don't want you to take clients away from them. That being said, I realized that if I was not going to receive help in building my business, I was going to need to rely on my intuition, my abilities, my work ethic and myself. What it comes down to is this: often times in becoming successful, you have to trust yourself. I call it relying on the spirit of God within me, but others may simply call it self-reliance. Either way, you have to trust in yourself, educate yourself and believe that you will succeed, all the while offering quality service.

My fears were many: fear of my wife not being taken care of, and fear that my business model wouldn't work in Central PA for a person of color. I had never been my own boss and had a big fear of the unknown. However, I ignored all of this and was so overwhelmed with the possibility of success, that I did not let my fears stop me. I was also being guided by what I believed my purpose as a father and husband was, which was to create an atmosphere where my kids could have access to me. That is another key element to my story: while fear may be real, we need to fix our eyes on the positive possibilities of making a leap of faith, rather than on the obstacles and fears that hold us in place.

I am thankful that this transition has created a space for my family and me to be fed. I am now able to have the mental space to make my girls and my wife more of a priority and walk more fully in my life's purpose.

When I think about redefining the word "profit," in the general sense, profit occurs when a transaction takes place, and something positive is left over as a result. When I made a transaction with God to say that I was going to leave my career as an educator and move in the direction of taxes and financial advising, the profits I experienced were many. Personally, the profits are both financial and spiritual. In terms of others, my wife and children are profiting by having me more available to meet their needs. The community I am serving is profiting by having a service available to them, and an advisor who cares about providing them quality work. There has been so much profit in so many areas that I really believe it is because of my jumping out into the unknown, pursuing a life of passion and redefining what profit means.

Walking away from this story, it is important to know that there is so much profit when you find your purpose. There is profit in the financial sense but it can also be spiritual, emotional and psychological. The community around you can profit when you walk in your purpose, as well as your family, friends and loved ones. It includes emotionally stability, an eagerness to see life in a positive way and a desire to see people and communities changed for the better. My hope is that after reading this, people will be motivated to reassess their lives and to see where they can more fully walk out their purpose. If you can find your life's work to be closely tied to whatever that purpose is, I can almost guarantee that profit, in all of its forms, will come.

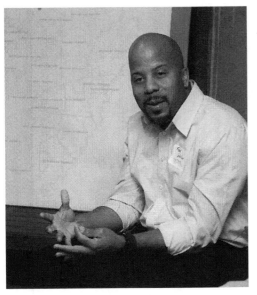

Fred Waller is an entrepreneur, published author, and workshop facilitator. He is the owner of Waller Tax and Financial. He received his BSE in Mathematics from Millersville University. After leaving teaching, he opened up his Financial Services firm time. He owns and operates a financial services firm providing tax investment and insurance services to both individuals and small businesses. He eventually earned the status of Enrolled Agent with the Internal Revenue Service and Certified Financial Planner (CFPO)

In addition to being an entrepreneur, Fred is a Deacon at Bright Side Baptist Church in Lancaster, Pa and teaches both Noon Day and 7:00 pm Bible Study. Fred is also a community minded person. He is a Crown Financial Ministries Budget Coach. In 2011, Fred was a recipient of the Cornelius Award that identifies, "A God-Fearing Man, Respected by His Community". Fred is also a member of Alpha Phi Alpha Fraternity Incorporated.

Fred is the author of the book, "The Truth Shall Set Your Free: Biblical Truths That Reveal God's Plan for Financial Freedom". Fred uses this book for workshop facilitation as well in Philadelphia and Central Pa area for many years.

When Fred isn't' helping his clients or teaching, he enjoys golf and creating memories with his family.

Fred currently resides in Lancaster, Pa with his wife Lynette, their two children; Cheyanne and Kylee and their dog Chip.

Fred can be reached at www.wallertax.com

Movement IS Medicine

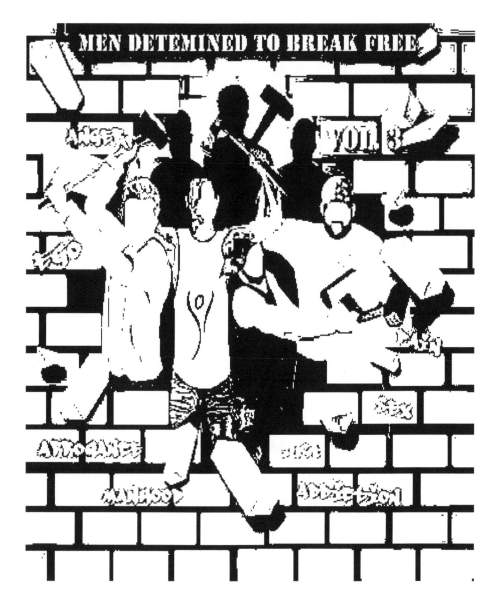

Chapter Nine

Overcoming Miscarriage
By
J. Marcellus Lynch

Fatherhood is one of the toughest yet most rewarding roles that God has blessed me with. My daughter, Jordan, turns eight this year and she is the epitome of a "Daddy's girl." It's hard to believe that not so long ago I was in a place where I didn't think I would ever be a father. Our struggle to become parents was the most emotionally draining, mentally taxing ordeal that I have ever dealt with. My wife and I suffered through a total of five miscarriages during our eighteen years of marriage. Although we are parents now, that ordeal still has a hold on certain parts of my life.

Being a father was something I figured would come easy. I always assumed that my biggest battle would be becoming a great father. I was the youngest of seven children with a really large family on both sides. There were many examples in my life of men who epitomized what it means to be a great father, so the bar was extremely high. I admired my dad for the many ways that he modeled the definition of fatherhood. He was a very strong man in terms of his faith and his love for God and family. He had the greatest work ethic that I have ever witnessed and he showed me what it meant to be reliable whenever I committed myself to something. He was also a quiet man and had a sensitive side to him. He always expressed his love to me even when it came to discipline. In addition to my father's influence, all of my big brothers were parents by the time I got out of high school so I couldn't wait for my turn.

I actually almost became a father in my senior year of high school but my girlfriend at the time decided to have an abortion without letting me know. I had mixed feelings about it because I wasn't sure if the child was mine or the ex-boyfriend I was sure she was also still seeing at that time. Looking back on it now, I guess at that young age, it just wasn't my time to be a father. We were still together when I left for college but our relationship had ended during that summer. It wasn't long after that I met my wife, Erika, on the campus of Millersville University.

It was the summer of 1989 when I met Erika. She actually thought I was the boyfriend of a mutual friend who had come up to visit. We would later meet up at a campus party and never look back. She was someone who shared the same values ideals and goals as mine, as far as having a family. We both loved kids and came from very tight knit families. She was on the same page as me with wanting about three kids. We dated for several years, as we both got accustomed to being around each other's families. We were married in 1998 and were ready to embark on the life we both had talked about for years when we dated. We were both very excited about becoming parents. It was very important to both of us to deliver a grandchild to our parents. It's not that they didn't have any grandchildren but we were both the youngest of our siblings and we knew our parents couldn't wait to welcome the growth of our own family. Little did we know what we would go through before we reached that point.

In 2001, we went through the first miscarriage. We weren't ready for it. I don't think many new parents pay much attention to the risks that come with pregnancy. I had no idea that about 29% of pregnancies end in miscarriage. It was those kind of statistics that I paid a lot of attention to when the second pregnancy came around. I am thankful for the family and friends who were there to help us during that time period. It was truly a blessing. With all of help and support, I found most of the attention went to my wife at the time. Even I was careful to make sure I was there for her. Miscarriage is a terrible thing for a woman to go through. It wasn't about me. Later I would come to realize it was about me, too. Most men tend to internalize their feelings and not let them out so healing can begin. I was one of those men.

The second pregnancy was one of the hardest for me. I was not as excited as I was the first time. I had more feelings of apprehension than of joy, but these feelings were kept on the inside. On the outside, I was trying my best to be positive. Growing up in the church I knew I had to have faith. We made it almost to the exact point as the first pregnancy. I was stuck in the movie Groundhog Day. As the ultrasound technician maneuvered the instrument around my wife's belly the heartbeat we had witnessed at the last appointment had faded away. Again. This time I had to watch my wife pass the baby as if she had given birth in our bathroom. I would not wish that experience on my worst enemy. Life at that point felt unfair than it had ever been to me. I felt like God had pulled my chair from under me again.

After the second loss, I felt more left out during the grieving period. The calls were coming in but they were more focused on how my wife was doing. It was obvious she had to be going through more than I was, being the one who went through the physical loss, but what about me? I lost a child, too. It took me years to finally share what I was going through. I was too afraid of being called selfish and appearing weak. We would go through more losses over the next couple of years, and I was totally removed from any sense of joy in my life. On the outside, I'm sure I played my part but on the inside, I was going through a wave of depression. Most of my family and my friends probably never even realized it. My list of friends during that time was very short and the ones who I thought were friends weren't there for me. I felt like God wasn't there for me either. I was engaged in ministry and involved in my church but on the inside, I was growing apart from God. It was more about keeping myself busy so I would appear to be stronger than I was and free from the actual state of depression I was in at the time. I would continue to try to keep my head up and push through the season I was in after dealing with the four losses. My focus was my family and my church.

Movement IS Medicine

The holiday season was quickly approaching in 2006, when my father went into the hospital for a stress test. The doctor had some concerns regarding some blockage, and decided my dad needed a stint. The surgery went well and he was a few days away from going to a rehab facility. We were heading to a–retirement home to sing some Christmas carols after church when the hospital called to tell us to come there. My father was having a heart attack. We rushed there and were greeted by a nurse who immediately burst into tears. As my dad was getting his daily exercise, walking around the nurse's station, he had a massive heart attack. He was gone. Just like that. Just a few days before he was fine but apparently the stint had slipped and the blockage had worsened. We spent some time in the room with him as I made a bunch of calls to share the news about my father. Another loss.

My wife pulled me aside the day of my father's funeral to tell me she was pregnant again. Surely, this time it was meant to be right? It seemed God had taken my dad and delivered to us the child that we had always longed for. We decided to share the news despite our rule of waiting like the last two pregnancies. It was easier that way. Sometimes I felt that telling people about Erika being pregnant and then weeks later sharing the loss was becoming harder for them than it was for us. We tried so hard to be excited this time. We made it to that infamous appointment about thirteen weeks in and it resulted in the same experience. Another loss. I was starting to believe that fatherhood was just not in the books for me. It took me a while to think otherwise.

My relationship with my wife suffered in a lot of ways during this time. Intimacy was something I ran from over and over again. I shared with a marriage counselor one day that I saw intimacy as death. Every time we shared a moment of intimacy, the end result was death so I chose to not put myself in that position again. This caused many problems in our relationship. I refused to talk to anyone at this point. I was tired of talking about it. I took after my dad, who was a man of few words when it came to confronting issues. This drove my wife absolutely crazy. She was the complete opposite.

The weight issues stemming from the depression was another issue that had taken a serious toll on me. I had allowed myself to gain weight continuously to the point where my health was starting to take a turn for the worse. It was almost like the wait to becoming a father had affected the physical weight through the depression I was dealing with. I have always been a big guy but the last few years even after Jordan had come into our lives I was still going through a struggle with my weight. It wasn't until the Spring of 2015 that I decided to make a lifestyle change and start to do something about my physical state. I had simply had enough. With much support from family and friends I was able to not only lose 45 pounds but also accomplish a goal of running my first 5K event. Losing that weight helped me shed some of the mental and emotional strongholds that were keeping me down for so long.

One of the things that I had to deal with was I was becoming short tempered with people. The resentment I had for others who didn't take care of their kids. That was very difficult for me to see. How could they take being a parent for granted? God really had to deal with me on this. There was a girl who went to our church who had just had a baby. I didn't really know her story at the time but just knew she had a lot of kids and a few of them had been taken away from her by the state. Her newborn was the cutest baby ever. I would see my wife holding her and wished that God would one day bless us with a beautiful child like her.

We started to talk about adoption and had taken some classes back when we had taken our nephew in with us for a short period. I was always open to adoption as an option, even if we had never had a miscarriage. The thought of being there to take care of a child that had no one there for them was a beautiful thing. Months later, we were contacted through an agency about a child who was recently separated from her parents. The agency was given our name by the baby's mother. The same baby I had previously viewed my wife holding in church was the one we received the call about. After many calls and visits with the agency they set up a visit with the child who was at a foster home not far from us. We bonded right away with her. She was around 18 months old when she came to stay with us for a weekend visit. I was returning from visiting family in North Carolina, while my wife stayed behind to get some things ready for the visit. That visit ended up being the first of a few visits, and before long she would come to stay with us for good.

God had finally blessed us. It's hard to believe that the same little girl that my wife sometimes held in church is now our daughter. In spite of all of the losses and all the tears that we shed, we are finally parents. It was and still is an awesome feeling. It is everything I have wished for and dreamed about. There are still some things I need to work out in order to get back to the place where I once was with my wife.. The scars of miscarriage are tough ones to deal with, even for men. However, I do know that God is able. This is why I stated that fatherhood is one of the toughest roles I have ever had.

There is no other option for me but to be the best father that I can be to my daughter. She deserves that. Every time I hear her call out to me, whether it is to greet me as I enter the house from a long day at work, or when she cries out to me when she is distressed or upset, I think about the times when I wasn't sure if I would ever have those moments. My current experiences as a father have helped to ease some of the pain from our many losses. However, I have to be honest and admit that the healing process is complicated, as the past cannot be fully erased. Regardless, I am glad that I never fully gave up on fatherhood, as it is one of the most important roles that I have been blessed with in this life.

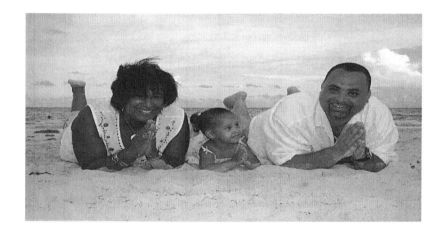

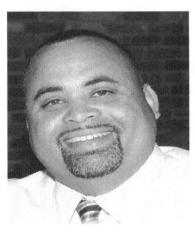

J. Marcellus Lynch is a native of Philadelphia, currently residing in Coatesville Pa., with his wife Erika and their 7-year-old daughter Jordan. He was brought up through the Philadelphia School System graduating from R.E. Lamberton H.S. and also attended Millersville Univ. of PA. He's currently seeking a B.S. in Photography and works hard balancing family and serving Christ at Mt. Zion Baptist Church in Coatesville.

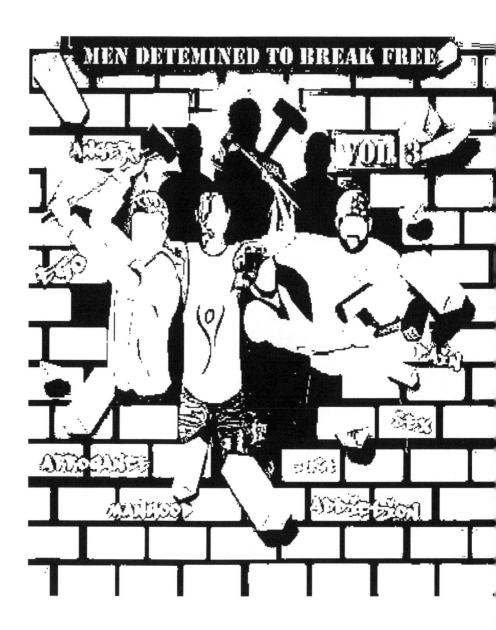

Chapter Ten
#Hopegiver
By
Chris M. McNeil

My name is Christopher McNeil and my hope is that reading my story will help you to overcome the obstacles in your life. I grew up on the corner of Beaver and Andrew Streets in Lancaster, Pennsylvania with my grandmother and my mother and lived there from the age of two until I was twenty-four. Both of these strong Black women were intent to have my siblings and I receive a good education. My grandmother was my first hope-giver. She had a third grade education but read the Bible to me every morning and as a result of this intervention, I was reading by the age of two. She was born in South Carolina and stopping school to help out on the farm where she grew up on. Her mother died very young and her father was unknown. Her maternal grandfather was a Civil War veteran and her grandmother received a pension from the military. She lived with relatives and moved to Florida briefly then moved to Pennsylvania to work, live, and worship with Mennonite families. She stated in her later years that the Mennonites were the only people who accepted her for who she was. She could not write well and wrote her signature with the letter X. My mother was adopted at three days old in Philadelphia. Her birth mother is very much alive and has visited our home often. Her father is unknown to this day.

Movement IS Medicine

I am the product of an affair. My mother was a sophomore in high school when she became pregnant with me. My father was married and had a family in South Carolina. My sister was born two years later from the same relationship.

I never had a relationship with my natural father, who was killed in a car accident when I was six years old. I don't remember him, although I have heard that he was very handsome and all the women chased after him. He had a good job and when he passed away, he had earned enough Social Security and life insurance to take care of his four children.

I was born during the Hurricane Agnes flood in June of 1972, two months premature. My mother told me that the forces tried to stop me from entering the Earth. My umbilical cord was wrapped around my neck as I was being born. From day one, obstacles were in my way but I overcame them. I was a pleasant kid but deep down I was angry. In addition, I suffered abuse from a close family friend who is now deceased. Because of this, I felt timid, fearful, and mistrusting. I was mad, frustrated, disappointed and above all, I felt abandoned. I got all failing grades in school, barely graduating from high school. I failed to apply myself in the classroom even though I was more than capable.

I struggled with confidence and it showed up in many areas of my life. I refused to play sports and athletics during school. I was forced to fulfill an inappropriate role for a child due to the absence of a true natural father. There are many Black males living in homes without a fatherly presence, due to abandonment and incarceration. I had to be the "man of the house." I was the protector and my mother was the provider, sometimes working two jobs while she earned her education at night, making the honor roll and getting A's. This inappropriate role caused me to grow up much faster than others. I was dropping off the rent, cable, buying groceries and preparing meals for the family while my mother worked.

As a result of my upbringing, I was a bitter young man. I smiled a lot to cover my inner rage; meanwhile all hell was breaking loose inside me. At times, I didn't express my emotions in the best way. I had issues with male authority figures and anger on the job when a person in authority that didn't look like me redirected me. I can recall a time when I became so angry with my supervisor that I put window cleaner in his soda and put it back in the refrigerator. I tried to hurt him.

I would attempt to abuse animals and dream about hurting people and babies. I would break windows and lie compulsively. I was beginning to associate with the wrong crowds for attention. The jail cell and the casket were awaiting me although my behavior in school was acceptable. The crowd I was associating with was not good and if I was not cautious, I would become just like them. However, I was good at being deceptive and making others feel comfortable while maintaining my agenda.

I was always searching for that father figure and my mother put me in salient church programs, the Boy Scouts and Teen Haven where I met many strong, solid Christian men who genuinely cared for me. It was a learning experience for me because it kept me out of trouble and on the right track but there was something still missing. As an adult, I worked as an Urban Outreach Project Specialist for the Boy Scouts of America and as a counselor for Teen Haven, and as a Sunday School teacher for every church where I have been a member. Paying it forward is important for our populations.

I didn't have a father to show me how to become a man. After graduating from junior college, I won several college scholarships for basketball and thought that dating several young ladies and all that goes with being an athlete would fill the emptiness NOPE!

I thought parties would fill the void, NOPE! I thought marrying a wife, buying a home, having children, would fill the void. Nope!! Even with church, there was still a void.

I thought that getting an awesome grade point average in graduate school would help but that still wasn't the answer, my life was full, yet empty. I was a cracked egg!!! All those successes were like putting Band-Aid's on cracked eggs. I was still bleeding from a wound that would not heal. I came to a crossroads in my life. Either break the dysfunctional cycle or blaze a new trail.

Then a few years ago, a friend told me that unless I allowed God to father me I would continue to stay stuck and to spin my wheels. I never realized that God was there the whole time when my biological father did not bother to acknowledge my existence.

Once I allowed God to father me, my life was incomplete. However, He filled the void, healed the heartache and today I am free from anger, frustration, abandonment, disappointment and fatherlessness and now I have five beautiful children with a beautiful wife who I have been with over half of my life. Now I am able to help counsel others using my pain.

In 2011, I began an educational odyssey that was very profound. In August of that year, I was accepted into graduate school at Lincoln University of Pennsylvania with a concentration in counseling/psychology. I figured that I would take my pain and heartache and help others heal. The first semester was a learning experience, but I earned a 3.3 GPA. The next semester, I earned a 3.75 GPA, and lost my job the next day. That experience taught me that everyone patting you on your back isn't for your benefit. God has definitely ordered my steps. I applied for a job at a local community center as an Outreach Specialist, which was a salaried position, perfect for that time in my life. I earned my graduate degree because someone said I could do it. I attended classes where the professors looked like me and had PhD's. It's important to surround ourselves with dreamers and people who can pour goodness into our lives. We also have to seek professional help when we suffer from traumatic experiences. Victory over our issues symbolizes hope and builds faith. It gives hope for the hopeless. If you start out with less than favorable conditions, that doesn't mean you will end up there.

Now, since graduating with my Masters' degree, I've become a mentor to others going through the Masters program. Professionally, I am a therapist working toward becoming a Licensed Professional Counselor and opening my own counseling agency. I will begin matriculation toward my doctoral degree this fall. I am also a facilitator of an empowerment and awareness program called

Project 180, which addresses dysfunction in families and helps those who are focused on becoming successful in spite of the absence of their fathers from their lives.

My pain transformed my purpose and I was able to let go of the anger I had! Someone gave me hope! I'm thankful for the people who gave me hope and who gave me encouragement. I aim to do the same to others that need my encouragement. Hope never dies but the heart can become sick sometimes when hope is deferred.

Christopher M. McNeil
#hopegiver

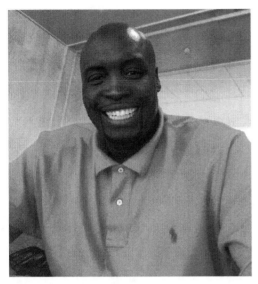

Chris McNeil is a Masters' Level Clinician in the Richmond, VA area, relocating to the area in 2014. His clients include adults and children with multiple diagnoses ranging from schizophrenia, Bipolar Disorder, ADHD, Oppositional Defiant Disorder to name a few.

A Lancaster, Pennsylvania native, Chris earned his Master of Science in Human Services-Counseling in 2013 from The Lincoln University of Pennsylvania. Chris is currently matriculating through post-Masters coursework toward licensure as a licensed professional counselor (LPC). He is scheduled to begin his doctorate (Ed.D) coursework at Fielding Graduate University in Fall of 2016. He is the founder of Project 180, an empowerment and awareness program for the fatherless and travels to lecture and bring awareness to the issues of dysfunctional families. Chris also volunteers at several juvenile detention centers in the area, empowering youth to make good choices.

He is writing a book titled, "Learn, Heal, Love, We learn from the past, we heal in the present, we love going forward".

Chris is married to his wife of 18 years, Terry, and they have 5 children ages 10 to 21.

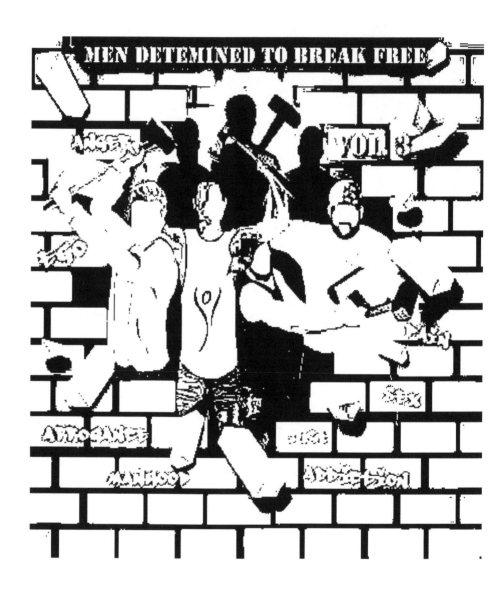

Chapter Eleven
One Man's Mission to Pay It Forward
By
Donnell Regusters

I was born in Southwest Philadelphia and raised in the nearby suburb of Yeadon, Pennsylvania. I had the privilege of living in the city with family then moving to this suburb right outside of Philadelphia. So, I was able to experience city life with the comfort of suburban living. That's not to say that my life was perfect by any means but I have always had a great mother and good role models in my life. When I was young in the mid-1980s, like many other Black people who had the means, my mother decided to move out of the inner city. Crack was ravishing cities all over the country and Philadelphia was not immune. I remember the crack era and the victims of that urban crisis. They were not just the addicts but innocent individuals like Marcus Yates, a young boy caught in the crossfire of bullets in the city. I remember people being robbed and shot for their Jordan's'. They would hand them over and still get shot. I remember the MOVE bombing and I watched the smoke from my apartment in Yeadon when I was eight years old. This is the context of the times and the city that I come from. The crazy thing is that it doesn't feel like much has changed. That is why I find it a necessity in life to "Pay it Forward." I have experienced ups and downs in life and I understand the environment many of the young people that I mentor come from. I feel a need and a duty to be a part of helping young people in any way I can because there were people who believed in me. I know I could have easily been Marcus Yates just like many of us today know our kids could have met the same fate as Trayvon Martin.

I always knew from a young age that I wanted to be part of a movement or revolution for my people but I never knew what my role would be. Listening to Public Enemy and KRS-1 in my youth inspired me to recognize that I had a duty to help others. I found myself immersed in hip-hop culture and writing and wanting to learn film. A big influence on me was journalist Bonz Malone, one of the best music journalists of his time. I began to understand that my art could be a part of how I became involved in the growth of my community. Telling our stories is important. I began writing and interviewing artists during the '90s hip-hop era and then proceeded to film school. Now I work at telling our stories visually from documentaries to short interviews.

The film and media industry is not an easy business to work in. I had to find a way to support myself while embarking on the journey to become a filmmaker. I fell into teaching because a local charter school needed someone to teach film and video production. Teaching was the last thing I ever thought that I would do with my life but in all honesty, it has been the most rewarding thing I've ever done in my life. Many of my friends in the arts have found their way to education. The issues in our schools have made it necessary for independent artists to become involved with schools by setting up after-school programs or teaching classes during the day. Many schools have scrapped art and afterschool programs, so the community picks up where the schools district dropped off.

Mentoring has been something I have always done even when I didn't know it. I'm a natural teacher because I have an inquisitive nature and I like to share the things I learn with others it. If I know something cool, I automatically want other people to know it. I found that teaching life skills was my niche in education. My passion is in teaching young people the things like that will help them be able to function in society without giving up who they are on the inside. They are essential life skills like conflict resolution, job readiness, and anger management. I also taught the lessons that my mother taught me. For example, it's important to realize that life is all about the little things and it's not always what you say but how you say it.

The best part of teaching for me is witnessing the light bulb goes off in a person's mind. When I see that someone understands something that I taught them and then later uses it, I know I have done my job. For example, I enjoy teaching words that I know my students would never use unless they were exposed to them in my class. Then when they come back and use the word in front of me with a big smile on their faces, it just shows me the influence that I have on their lives. It also shows me that they enjoy learning even if they don't know it yet.

A good friend of mines once told me when I first started teaching that, "You are going to lose some." I took that in and understood it but didn't fully grasp it until it happened. When it happened to me personally, it rocked me. Living in a city like Philadelphia when you hear someone has died, the first thing that pops into your head is that they were murdered. That is a part of the mentality of city living because there is so much violence. In order for me to rationalize the deaths of the young people in my life, I thought, "well at least none of them were murdered." I don't like thinking that way but I had to make myself come to grip with their deaths somehow. One of my students died in a car accident, the other passed away in her sleep and the third died from an aneurism. In addition, I have one young man in prison. Their peers and teachers alike loved them all. I still think of them often. Sometimes I'll remember a joke they told a story or me about their life. I didn't attend any of the funerals of my students that passed away. I had my own personal cry for them and I kept to myself. On the surface, I really don't know why I didn't go. I could have gone but I did not. When I really look inside of my thoughts, I don't think I was ready to see them in a box. Who is ready to see anyone that they have known lying in a casket? It's the one place we know we will all end up. The only thing is you don't expect people younger than you to be laid to rest before you.

When I stopped teaching I began mentoring and organizing young people around the city regarding education reform. It's one thing for adults to speak up for their kids but it's another thing when you hear young people speaking to empower and fight for their rights in school. I recruited young people and met with them afterschool to prepare and to educate them on the issues. I learned a lot from the young people I have taught and mentored. I think the biggest lesson I learned is that you have to reach people where they are and you can't force your expectations on them. You can set high standards for them to achieve but they have to find their own path, no matter how much you want them to walk the paths you have laid out for them.

In conclusion, throughout my life as an educator and mentor, I have recognized a glaring omission to the community. We need more men involved in the community and/or teaching in the classrooms. That's not to say that there aren't good men doing that work now. The point is that we are having so many problems that we need all hands on deck. People don't need to be full time teachers. They just need to be involved in more than the lives of their own children. Find the time to mentor and model the things that make you a respectable person, talented artist/ businessperson or a great parent. Those influences are needed by our young people in order to help them to make the most of their lives.

Donnell Regusters is a media professional who began his career as a journalist while he was a student at the University of Maryland at College Park. He began working at Comcast where he produced news segments for the public affairs department. Working on news segments and projects like the critically acclaimed Paper Chasers Hip Hop Documentary he learned how to produce. Donnell began interviewing talent on camera and produced segments for a TV show called Hip-Hop Nation that was syndicated throughout the country on NBC. While producing his own work and writing screenplays he produced segments and worked for Back 2 Basics Real Rap TV one of Philadelphia's premier hip-hop shows. He has worked as an advocate for education reform, teacher, and mentor to Philadelphia youth while working as a freelance photographer and videographer.

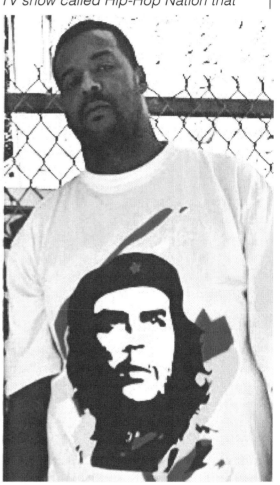

Movement IS Medicine

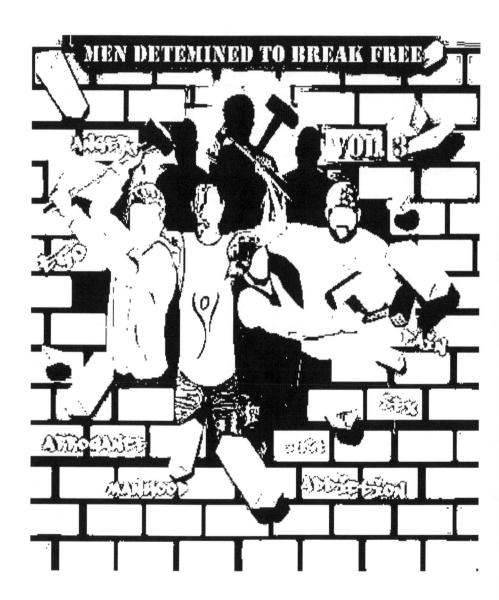

Chapter Twelve
But God
By
Al B. Quarles II

"He sent out his word and healed them; he rescued them from the grave." ~Psalm 107:20

Let me start by saying that I can honestly never remember a time in my life when I did not know that Jesus existed, loved me, responded to my prayers, and that I had a special purpose on this earth, that only He would slowly reveal.

Like most men, the concept of seedtime and harvest never truly resonates when it comes to the many things that we put our mind, body, and spirits through. For me, it was mainly my body. I think that when it comes to our health, as men, we just do not want to know or hear any unfavorable reports, so we bury our heads in the proverbial sand, and stay away from the healthcare system as much as possible.

I decided that 2015 would be my year to place my health at the forefront of my existence. After all, I was 47 years old with a new wife, a new baby boy bearing my name, two beautiful daughters, normal aches, pains, and an occasional bloody stool during bowel movements that I saw as my only health concern. I pushed it to the back of my mind and it would always eventually go away.

Overall, I considered myself healthy even though I didn't practice clean eating. I knew that one day I would turn that corner and join many of my friends on their quest to obtain and maintain good health. Until then, most things that I needed to address medically I could find on WEBMD, and through other Internet research that would inevitably lead me to misinformation. I was even able to convince my primary care doctor whom I had only seen twice in several years, of my self-diagnosis of hemorrhoids. When I finally

144

scheduled that appointment for an annual physical exam, it was far past due.

As I was about to leave the appointment, my doctor also recommended that I needed to get a colonoscopy due to my age, and referred me to specialist. I was thinking, this is not cool, not needed, and they are not going to violate this Black man right here! .... especially since I was not yet 50 years old.

I avoided seeing a specialist for several weeks and continued with the home remedies, over the counter medications and my faltering prescription medication given by my doctor, until all of these things finally aided in my situation getting worse. One positive thing I can say I did was to make sure to stay at the altar for prayer at church. I had all of my deacons and my pastors praying for me, and even though I was not certain of what was going on, I needed to plant healing seeds in the ground, as well as touch and agree with like-minded individuals.

After more complications and another trip to my primary care doctor for a new and improved medication, I decided to man up and schedule an appointment with the colon and rectal specialist. My first visit was mainly painless. The first thing that the doctor did was praise me for coming. "I do not see nearly enough African American males in my office, and when I do, it is often too late. Tell your friends to come see me; it's really not that bad."

Time quickly passed and in a week, I found myself at the surgery center preparing for my colonoscopy. This was truly an easy procedure, and the worst part by far was drinking the prep and taking the required laxatives.

In the recovery room after the procedure, the doctor met with us and informed me that he found a polyp during the examination and took a biopsy to have it tested. Normally they remove polyps during the exam, and many of my friends informed me that they had the same tests done with no concern, so I did not worry about it. The doctor cleared me to go on my upcoming golf trip, saying he would talk to me when the results came back.

The hand of God then began to reveal itself to me in ways that were confusing but very real. From that day on I had begun to be awakened at night constantly hearing Jason Nelson's song entitled,

"I am", in my head. It also seemed to be playing every time I turned on the radio in my car. The part of the song that disturbed me was the line, "The doctor says cancer but... I AM." It continued repeatedly and even though I knew that the meaning was positive, the reality of the word cancer was a very alarming possibility. I informed my wife and mother that the song was driving me crazy, and I could not seem to shake it. Every morning at 4 A.M., I woke up to hear the song in my head. It got so bad that I stopped listening to my favorite gospel radio station in the car because I didn't want to hear the song anymore. What is God trying to say? Is he preparing me for a cancer diagnosis?

By this point, I had forty guys already registered for a golf trip I was coordinating for my golf club, "The Bogey Boyz." We were headed to Myrtle Beach, South Carolina for some rest, relaxation, and a great time. Even though I hadn't hit a golf ball all year because I didn't feel well enough to practice, as president of the club, I thought, "The show must go on."

After a few painful rounds of golf in Myrtle Beach and several Motrin 800's that I had begun to cherish and call "Chicklets", I was playing surprisingly well, and found myself in first place heading into our annual team tournament that Friday. I was working with the golf course pro and his staff to get us started that afternoon. I walked to my car to gather a few items, and my phone rang with a call from my doctor that changed my life forever.

"Hey Al, are you back from your golf trip yet?"

"No, we just got here the other day and we're actually just getting ready to tee off in our annual team tournament."

On Friday, May 1, 2015, my doctor informed me that they had found cancer cells in the biopsy and that I had colorectal cancer. "The doctor says cancer but... I AM." I did not hear much more during that conversation, but I somehow managed to remain calm as he said, "Just take one shot at a time, enjoy your trip, and I will see you when you get back." Even writing this now, I get chills.

The true testimony began at that moment. God had already prepared me to hear what the doctor was going to say with Jason Nelson's song, so now it was time for me to put my faith into action.

The first thing that I remember saying to myself is that I have believed in God all of my life for a reason, and this must be it.

"If thou faint in the day of adversity, thy strength is small."
~Proverbs 24:10

As I collected my thoughts and headed back to join my group I first ran into a good friend who was on the trip named Derrick. He was relaxing in his car and appeared to be waiting for me. I am not sure why I felt very comfortable sharing my recent diagnosis with him, but I immediately did. His response was simply, "Let's pray, my brother".

We stood in the parking lot and held hands as he began to pray aloud and declare healing and complete victory over my disease in Jesus name. I don't remember much of what was going on around us, but I am certain that several golfers coming from their cars had to think we were religious fanatics summoning the golf gods. But in that prayer I truly believed and received my healing at that moment. I promised myself that I would not worry, grow weak, or lose focus. I also decided that I was not going to own what the doctor had told me, and refused to even use the word cancer. It is actually strange for me even now to use it while penning this testimony. But that was the diagnosis they gave me: colorectal cancer.

After calls to my wife, sister, and pastor, I was even more encouraged because they all spoke life over me, instead of sympathy. They all encouraged and reinforced the prayer I shared with Derrick, and they all believed in and knew of the healing power of God. My pastor simply said, "Now you just have to walk this thing out".

I returned to the group, gave the final instructions for the tournament, and went out in the rain and shot the best golf score that I have ever shot in my entire life as I broke 80 for the first time. I shot a 78 while leading my team to win the tournament. I went on to win my club championship that Saturday.

And the peace of God, which passeth all understanding, shall keep your hearts and minds through Christ Jesus. ~Philippians 4:7

Meanwhile at home, life continued. My new wife, new baby boy, two daughters and mother still needed and depended on me as the man of the house. My job and the thousands of homeless and displaced students that I serve every year through my job with the School District of Philadelphia still needed me. My pastor asked me to order a series on healing by Pastor Creflo Dollar of World Changers Ministries, and the lessons immediately reinforced what I was learning at Higher Ground Church International. The spiritual foundation and scriptures, many of which I am sharing in this chapter set the tone and direction of my entire process. The significant message that continues to speak volumes to me is that our "faith" is what moves the hand of God. We have to stand on scriptures as our belief and foundation, and Jesus is the reason it is possible.

As I was gearing up for the fight of my life God was already working. In addition to allowing His great works, He had just given me a wife, who was my backbone; who would not allow me to speak anything but life. I don't think she will ever truly understand how much I appreciate her, but her strength was truly what I needed during those doubtful moments.

I talked to God frequently in prayer, and soon I knew that I needed a teaching hospital that was highly ranked and on the cutting edge of technology. I had to calm my emotions and listen to the ultimate doctor, and not just any doctor. I learned the importance of having a team that has seen as many cases and performed as many procedures as possible in a specific area of expertise. I learned this through consultation with my brother-in-law, a cancer surgeon at MD Anderson in Houston, Texas. Without my knowledge, my brother-in-law had begun polling his colleagues working in my specific area of oncology, and they all independent of each other, recommended that I meet with a specific surgeon at the Hospital of the University of Pennsylvania. The ironic twist was that since my brother-in-law had first become a urologic oncologist, I had always feared needing him for medical advice. However, when the day came,

Movement IS Medicine

I knew that it was definitely a blessing that God had planned ahead of the time.

And we know that all things work together for good to them that love God, to them who are the called according to his purpose. ~Romans 8:28

Once I met with my new surgeon and expressed my belief system and faith in God, I was completely reassured when she, unlike other doctors I had come in contact with, agreed with my beliefs, echoed my sentiments, encouraged my faith, and although she may not have completely understood, she told me that I would be ok. My spirit was definitely at ease with her, and like other situations that God revealed His hand in, it was seamless. Additional confirmation came when my Goddaughter, who is a nurse, randomly called me later that week and told me that she had performed the same surgical procedure with my surgeon on numerous occasions. My mind was at ease.

The plan for my medical treatment and ultimate healing included chemotherapy and radiation therapy running concurrently on Monday through Friday for six straight weeks. Time to heal would follow this, surgery to remove the polyp turned tumor, and then twelve more chemotherapy sessions occurring every other week for three straight months.

As I planned to move forward with my process, I needed the word of God daily because I needed to be less focused on my symptoms and more on my healing. I/we just cannot separate the two. I could not be swayed by unfavorable doctor reports when they came, unbelievers when they showed up, or what outcome may have happened to others in my situation. During this critical period in my life, I even had to change some of my friends. I could not hang around unbelievers who may have influenced me or encouraged doubt. Others seemed to stay away from me because they didn't know how to respond or what to say.

During my first radiation treatment, they asked if there was a special type of music that I liked. I said gospel, not thinking they could accommodate, but they managed to find a gospel CD in their collection. Thereafter, as soon as I walked into the radiation suite on following visits the staff automatically hit the play button and I heard gospel music during every single treatment for 6 weeks. The music and artists ministered to me on a daily basis.

In addition, the side effects of chemotherapy and radiation that they warned me about and monitored me for were almost non-existent other than occasional nausea and some skin discomfort from the radiation. I also believed in my heart and soul that I was getting better.

Following my abdominoperineal resection surgery, the hospital released me a week early because I responded and recovered so well. They also did a biopsy of the material collected during the operation and tested 16 lymph nodes. The pathology report stated that they could not find one trace of cancer in any of the specimens. "Sixteen lymph nodes, negative for carcinoma." They found that I was a "total response" to chemotherapy and radiation. My surgeon said, "We are extremely pleased. You did great. Your results are not typical." After reviewing my final report, my brother-in-law who has seen thousands of cancer patients called it "miraculous." The reality of my situation was that even before they removed the area where they initially had found cancer, there was no cancer any longer. It was already gone. It may sound crazy and people can believe whatever they want to believe, but I know what it was.

When I had a follow up visit after a month of recovery, I met with my oncologist and she immediately hugged me. She continued to tell me how pleased she was with how well I responded to my treatment and on the following visits, she expressed how she had been deeply concerned for my family and me when I first presented. "You were very sick. I was very concerned for you and your family. I am so happy for you." I really hadn't known how bad it was until that moment. On one of our last visits during my precautionary chemotherapy sessions, she came into the room to see me and even shed a tear when she was leaving the examination room.

Jesus said unto him, If thou can believe, all things are possible to him that believeth.
~Mark 9:23

I have since finished all of my treatment and recovery. My testimony goes far beyond this story, and has so many details that I will definitely need to one day write my own full-length book in order to give a full account of the wonders and ways that God has blessed me and my family throughout this storm. I only wanted to capture the essence of my story in hopes that it will encourage and bless someone.

My hope is that as a result of this story, Black men will go to their doctors more frequently when they have a concern, and not wait until after a simple cure or procedure is no longer possible. When caught early, even cancer can be handled fairly easily. I also hope that every Black man age 45 and older gets a colonoscopy in order to have peace of mind, and also taste the wonders of Propofol (I'm only serious). But even more importantly, I hope that all of us realize how powerful faith is. I put mine to the test and once again, God has never failed. Not even once.

Movement is Medicine

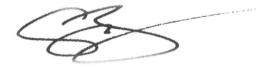

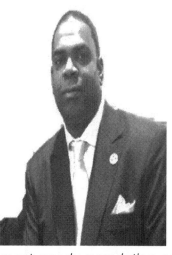

Al B. Quarles, II, M. Ed., was born and raised in Abington, Pennsylvania, and is a graduate of Abington Senior High School. He also has attended Millersville University of PA, where he earned a Bachelor of Science Degree, and Temple University, where he earned a Master Degree in Educational Psychology.

Mr. Quarles currently works as an administrator for the School District of Philadelphia, and serves as the Philadelphia Coordinator of the Education of Children and Youth Experiencing Homelessness Program. While diligently working to serve the most needy population of students in Philadelphia, Mr. Quarles has been appointed on two occasions and currently serves on the Pennsylvania Secretary of Educations Homelessness Task Force, is the author of the highly acclaimed Burning Sands literary series, and has over 20 years experience as an administrator, counselor, and behavioral health professional working with children.

Al is a charter member of the Abington-Ambler Alumni Chapter of the Kappa Alpha Psi Fraternity Incorporated, the proud founder of the multiple award winning Bogey Boyz Golf Club and "Bogey Kids" Junior Golf Mentoring Program for under-privileged youth in Philadelphia and Montgomery Counties. Al is a proud husband and father of three, who is always looking to serve those less fortunate than himself especially children who, he feels, are the most vulnerable in society today. Al can be reached at Abquarles2@gmail.com

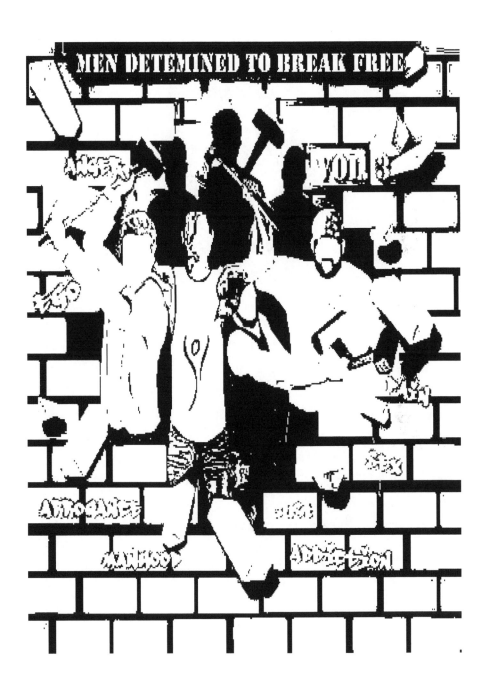

Notes from Assistant Editor
Adrienne Nolan-Owens

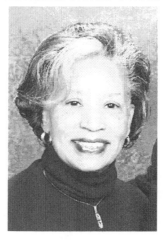

When Ramona Gaines asked me to do some editing for her books, without hesitation I said, "Sure!" I was happy to make a contribution to these projects. I love the written word, both reading and writing it. Perhaps it was because I had a hand in editing more of the chapters, that I felt a greater connection to this book. Or maybe it was reading these very personal stories written by men, who in my experience find it more difficult than women, to openly express deep feelings. Their narratives of moving past pain and suffering, through growth and development, to peace and fulfillment were inspiring. God's grace and mercy was woven throughout many of them. I was truly moved by their stories, and hope they will have a positive impact on other men who read them. I feel privileged and blessed to have contributed to the final product.

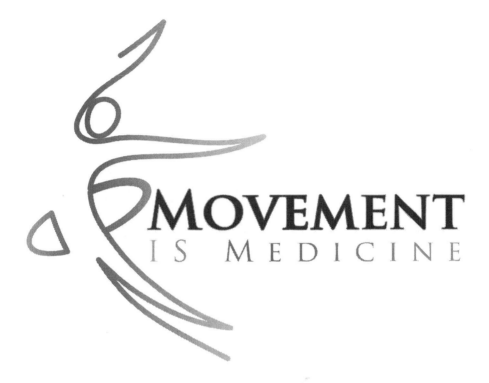

History

Movement IS Medicine is movement that was birthed to support you in honoring your body as a temple and doing what is necessary to achieve your goal to become whole.

And when He saw them, He said, " Go show yourselves to the priests."
And as they went they were healed
Luke 17:14

Movement IS Medicine Anthologies came about when founder Ramona M. Gaines started journaling about her weight loss on Facebook. The name Movement IS Medicine came from a conversation on Facebook with David Rosario one morning while sharing her morning meditations with friends. As her journals began to take shape the Lord led her to put it into book format. While she

155

was in the process of doing so others came along and began to share their stories with her either publicly on Facebook or inbox them privately. It was as if the Lord was using them to say this book is going to write itself if you don't come on and get it done. So Ramona sent out invitations to 25 women, 16 including her ended up in the finished product and that is how Movement IS Medicine Volume 1 was born. We knew that it would not just be one so that is why we decided to use the word Anthology.

Mission

Our mission is to empower God's people to take back their life one step at a time: to move God's people into a place of not just healing but wholeness. These goals will be achieved by sharing healthy recipes, exercising tips, and words of encouragement and inspiration to help and support you while on your own personal journey virtually. In addition to the virtual support we also provide in person support groups to come together to discuss "What's Eating You"? We understand that exercise and diet are key factors in a having a healthy lifestyle, but we also acknowledge that one's mental and emotional well-being are also important and does effect how we treat our temple.

For more information you may contact us at movementismedicine23@gmail.com

Follow us on Facebook, Twitter, Instagram and Pintrest

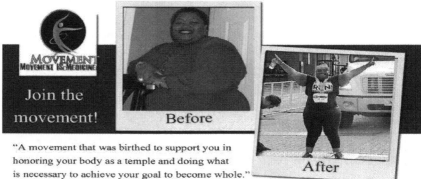

Join the movement!   Before

"A movement that was birthed to support you in honoring your body as a temple and doing what is necessary to achieve your goal to become whole."

movementismedicine23@gmail.com

After

Movement IS Medicine

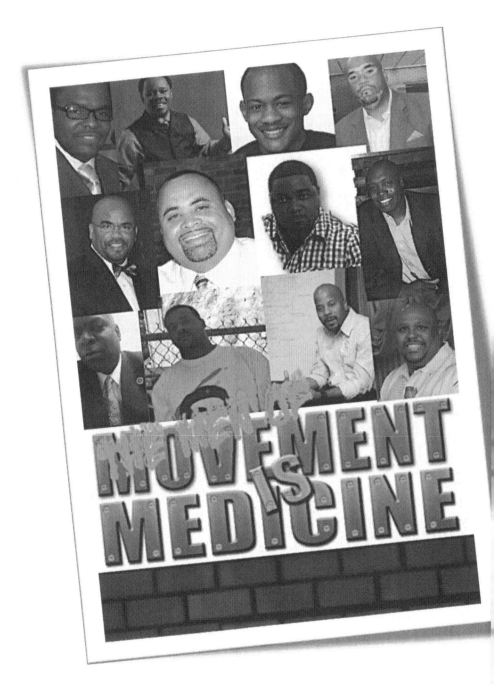

Movement IS Medicine

Made in the USA
Middletown, DE
28 September 2016